DATE

SEX, DIET, AND DEBILITY IN JACKSONIAN AMERICA

Contributions in Medical History
Series Editor: John Burnham

WOMEN & MEN MIDWIVES
MEDICINE, MORALITY, AND MISOGYNY IN EARLY AMERICA
Jane B. Donegan

AMERICAN MIDWIVES
1860 TO THE PRESENT
Judy Barrett Litoff

SPEECH AND SPEECH DISORDERS IN WESTERN THOUGHT BEFORE 1600
Ynez Violé O'Neill

SEX, DIET, AND DEBILITY IN JACKSONIAN AMERICA

SYLVESTER GRAHAM and HEALTH REFORM

STEPHEN NISSENBAUM

Contributions in Medical History, Number 4

GREENWOOD PRESS

WESTPORT, CONNECTICUT • LONDON, ENGLAND

Library of Congress Cataloging in Publication Data

Nissenbaum, Stephen.
  Sex, diet, and debility in Jacksonian America.

  (Contributions in medical history ; no. 4 ISSN
0147-1058)
  Bibliography: p.
  Includes index.
  1. Health attitudes—United States—History—19th
century. 2. Graham, Sylvester, 1794-1851.
3. Reformers—United States—Biography. 4. Grahamites.
5. Diet—United States—History—19th century.
6. Sex customs—United States—History—19th century.
7. United States—Social conditions—To 1865. I. Title.
II. Series.
RA418.3.U6N57   301.5   79-8280
ISBN 0-313-21415-8

Library of Congress Catalog Card Number: 79-8280
ISBN: 0-313-21415-8
ISSN: 0147-1058

First published in 1980

Greenwood Press
A division of Congressional Information Service, Inc.
88 Post Road West, Westport, Connecticut 06881

Printed in the United States of America

10 9 8 7 6 5 4 3 2 1

For JUDY

CONTENTS

PREFACE

While the focus of this book is on one man, Sylvester Graham, its purpose is somewhat broader. Graham was the first writer to formulate a coherent physiological analysis of the various new anxieties about the human body that had emerged by the 1830s, and to propose a systematic regimen he believed would assuage them. Coming out of both the evangelical ministry and the temperance movement of the late 1820s, he had a direct and significant impact on the development of movements such as vegetarianism, phrenology, and water-cure, in addition to sexual reform. To study Sylvester Graham is to study Victorian physiological theory and practice in the very act of coming into being—as a complete ideological system governing every aspect of private routine. The existing literature on these subjects has generally approached them piecemeal, as part of the history of sex, or diet, or temperance. The narrowness of my focus has permitted me to look at a relatively diverse body of literature as part of a single ideological system, and to examine it in the process of its development.

I have studied the evolution of this ideological system both as an episode in the history of ideas and as an aspect of Jacksonian social history. In dealing with Sylvester Graham's ideas I have tried to examine them on their own terms—to read the medical literature that Graham himself read. Also, I have tried to reconstruct something of the intellectual process by which he assimilated this literature, fastening on certain points and ignoring others, putting together selected elements from British, French, and American medical theory of the eighteenth and early nineteenth centuries and adding some of his own, and finally devising a new synthesis—"The Science of Human Life," he called it—that seemed to explain the inner and outer world he had come to inhabit.

One of the central ideas of Graham's system, for instance, was the principle that *stimulation led to debility*—a reverse of the conventional notion that debility was caused by too little stimulation (not enough hearty food, perhaps) rather than too much. I have traced in some detail the way Graham derived this idea from the work of the eighteenth-century physician Benjamin Rush and the way he combined it with ideas he encountered in other sources, especially French physiological theory, to arrive at a rationale for temperance, a vegetarian diet, and sexual continence. I have tried to examine this process not only as a way of tracing the transmission and transformation of ideas but also as a way of understanding those elements in Sylvester Graham's personal history that prepared him to be receptive to the idea that "stimulation" was a source of disorder. Here, biography becomes a clue to the meaning of intellectual history.

By placing Graham's personal experience in the broader context of social change during the first third of the nineteenth century—the transformation of a rural subsistence economy into a capitalist marketplace—I have tried to indicate some ways in which Graham's life was representative of his generation and his region, and thereby to suggest why certain other Americans in the 1830s and later might have found his ideas so persuasive. Finally, by investigating the composition of the constituency for whom the Graham System had its greatest appeal, I have tried to suggest something about the complex connection between this ideological system and the development of the bourgeois personality in the Jacksonian period.

To Sylvester Graham himself, and to his early followers, the new physiology represented a creative effort to come to terms with a set of experiences for which traditional rules about private behavior were ceasing to be relevant. Only for subsequent generations would this physiology be something learned from parents, physicians, and schoolbooks. Because I have examined the new ideology at the moment of its emergence, and not as the conventional orthodoxy it would later become, I am perhaps more sympathetic to it than other historians have been, although I hope I do not have to add that my sympathy is not to be confused with agreement.

In any case, it is not historical to equate the consequences of a new ideology with the intentions that led people to devise or adopt it. Just because Grahamite physiology can be seen in retrospect as leading to the development of a powerful bourgeoisie, it does not follow that either

Graham or his followers used it for that purpose. For instance, the dietary and sexual regimen Graham recommended did lead to *minimal consumption* of food and *minimal expenditure* of semen. Both these practices did result in saving money and signalling the willingness to defer or deny sensory gratification. But Graham made it clear on a number of occasions that he was less fearful of the loss of semen than he was of sexual excitement itself—even in the absence of orgasm. It was stimulation, not seminal emission, that led to debility and disease.

My reading of Grahamite physiology strongly suggests that Graham formulated his ideas not as a way to adopt the values of the capitalist marketplace but as a way to deny their power—to devise what I have called a physiology of subsistence. It is no accident that Henry David Thoreau lived by a close approximation of the Graham System during the two years he spent at Walden Pond.

Similarly, while it is true that Victorian sexual ideology had the effect of intensifying the powerlessness of women in nineteenth-century society, it does not follow that this ideology was devised out of male fear of female sexuality or out of male desire to maintain hegemony over women. First, sexual anxiety was only a single component of Grahamism. The system encompassed a whole constellation of issues—diet, for instance—that were hardly related to male hegemony. It is clear, furthermore, that men who adopted the Graham System were trying to desensualize themselves as well as their women, and that they paid perhaps fully as great a price by doing so.

Finally, Victorian sexual ideology was something of a double-edged sword that women were able to use, and possibly did use, to attain some real measure of independence over their sexual and reproductive lives. Victorian sexual theory provided women, for the first time, with at least the ideological basis for assuming the power to veto, or even to initiate, sexual contact with their husbands. As Orson S. Fowler, a phrenologist and Grahamite, proclaimed in the 1840s, it was for women to be "the final umpire" in the bedroom. And, as the career of Mary Gove Nichols makes clear, it was only a short step from orthodox Grahamism to radical feminism.

Before 1970 little was written about changing sexual ideas in nineteenth-century America. The one important exception was Sidney Ditzion's *Marriage, Morals, and Sex in America,* a comprehensive but necessarily superficial survey of sexual theory from Benjamin Franklin in the mid-eighteenth century to Alfred Kinsey in the mid-twentieth.[1] Ditzion devoted fewer than ten pages to Sylvester Graham and those he influenced directly, a group Ditzion labeled "The Healthians." Other significant studies that dealt, at least in part, with Graham and his circle included Richard H. Shryock's 1931 article, "Sylvester Graham and the Popular Health Movement"[2] and William Walker's 1955 dissertation, "The Health Reform Movement in the United States, 1830-1870."[3] Both of these works effectively placed Graham in his institutional context, but they were more concerned with his role as a forerunner of progressive health reform than with the intellectual origins or social significance of his ideology in its own time.

In a more popular vein, Gerald Carson's history of the breakfast cereal industry, *Cornflake Crusade*,[4] and Grace Adams's and Edward Hutter's *The Mad Forties*[5] portrayed the ferment Graham helped to set in motion as an example of the absurd if rather quaint eccentricities that marked the underside of nineteenth-century reform. Only seven pages from Siegfried Giedon's fascinating *Mechanization Takes Command* give a picture of Sylvester Graham that begins to resemble the one found in this book. Giedon portrayed Graham neither as a precursor of modernity nor as a silly eccentric, but as a case study in resistance to the mechanization of food production.[6]

During the present decade, however, the history of sex, diet, and health suddenly became a subject of serious historical inquiry. Several lines of research have led to an outpouring of scholarly contributions to the subject. The history of sexuality and diet has now been accepted, for example, as an important aspect of the history of medicine. Periodicals in medical history have published important articles including Arthur N. Gilbert and H. Tristram Englehardt, Jr.'s essays on nineteenth-century ideas about masturbation, John R. Bett's article on exercise, and James C. Whorton's work on the physiological rationale for vegetarianism.[7] Work of this sort has taken these matters out of the realm of trivia or taboo and has shown that they can be profitably subjected to the same analytic scrutiny as other areas of the history of ideas. At the same time, books by Joseph Kett and William Rothstein have shown how the same matters can be seen as a chapter in the history of the professionalization of American health care in the nineteenth century.[8]

The history of sexuality has also benefitted from the burgeoning of
the new social history, with its concern for the "private side" of historical experience and the lives of ordinary people. For instance, the
study of historical demography—work begun by Yasukichi Yasuba on
the decline of the birth rate in the United States after 1800—has led
scholars such as J. R. Potter and Daniel Scott Smith to examine the
changes in sexual behavior that led to this decline and were important
elements in the constellation of social pressures leading to the formulation of Victorian sexual ideology.[9]

Other nineteenth-century social historians developed an interest in
that ideology through their investigation of other aspects of social reform, especially the abolitionist movement. Two recent and important
books on this subject, Ronald Walters's *The Antislavery Appeal* and
Lewis Perry's *Radical Abolitionism*, have dealt, from differing perspectives, with the importance of sexual concerns in the lives and ideas of
prominent abolitionists. Both men have gone on to deal even more directly with sexuality, Walters in his 1974 anthology, *Primers for Prudery*,
and Perry in his forthcoming biography of Henry C. Wright.[10] Other
biographical studies, such as Robert David Thomas's book on John
Humphrey Noyes, and Ronald Numbers's work on the life of the
Seventh-Day Adventist "prophetess" Ellen White, have discussed their
subjects' views on sex and diet with a seriousness that would have been
impossible for historians only a few years ago.[11]

Closely related to this kind of study has been the emergence of a body
of scholarship that is concerned with the relationship between ideology
and class structure in the nineteenth century and tends to assign particular importance to benevolent reform, evangelical Christianity, temperance, and occasionally to sexual self-control. One approach, typified
by the important work of Paul Faler on the industrialization of Lynn,
Massachusetts, has been to suggest that this constellation of reforms
served the interests of industrial capitalists who needed to impose habits
of regularity and discipline on a lax and potentially disruptive labor
force. A somewhat different approach, represented in the work of Peter
Cominos and Charles Rosenberg on sexuality and Joseph R. Gusfield on
temperance, has been the contention that the new reform ideology functioned less as a mechanism of social control than as a tool of social
aspiration—aspiration to a condition of bourgeois respectability that
could be both achieved and displayed by living a life of restraint and

self-discipline, thereby gaining the economic and social benefits that derived from the deference or the denial of various forms of sensual gratification.[12]

Finally, perhaps the single development in the 1970s that has generated the most fruitful work on the subject has been the increased interest in the history of women's experience. Much of this scholarship has focussed on the desexualization of women in the nineteenth century. The work of G. J. Barker-Benfield and of John S. and Robin M. Háller, for example, has argued that Victorian sexual ideology provided a means by which middle-class males were able to increase their hegemony over women, while scholars such as Nancy Cott, Linda Gordon, and Carroll Smith-Rosenberg have pointed to the ways that women were able to use this same ideology for their own purposes.[13] Except for Barker-Benfield's book, *The Horrors of The Half-Known Life*, however, this feminist history has not been especially concerned with the effects of that ideology on men themselves. That is the subject of this book.

The introductory chapter is an account of Graham's personal and professional career in the context of social change in the early nineteenth century, and with a special focus on his notorious interest in the proper preparation of bread—"Graham bread," as it came to be known. The second chapter introduces the sexual ideas articulated by Graham and other reformers in the 1830s, contrasting them with the less anxious attitudes of earlier generations of Americans. Chapters 3 through 5 deal with the major intellectual sources of Graham's physiological theories and with the impact of those sources on Graham's early days as a temperance lecturer. Chapters 6 through 8 examine, in chronological order and in some detail, the way Graham expounded his system to a national audience in the three major works he published during the 1830s, culminating in his two-volume *Lectures on the Science of Human Life.*

Chapter 9 describes the spread of Graham's ideas in the succeeding decades and examines the nature of the audience to which his ideas seemed to appeal. Finally, the book concludes with a discussion of the way Grahamite ideology so deeply permeated American culture that it was accepted even by sexual radicals, like Dr. and Mrs. Thomas Low Nichols, who wished to replace monogamous marriage with a system of free love.

I first became interested in this general area when I encountered the

writings of Dr. and Mrs. Nichols, sexual theorists of the 1850s who
suddenly converted to Roman Catholicism while running a free-love
community. I was amazed, first of all, that anyone in that era would
write as openly about sexuality as the Nicholses did. But, it also struck
me that their radicalism smacked strongly of the very prudery they
ostensibly were protesting and that this paradox somehow made more
comprehensible their religious conversion and subsequent retreat into
conventional sexual morality. I felt the need to pursue the problem to
its origin, and this quest soon led me to Sylvester Graham—a figure
whose work proved central not only to the strange career of Mary Gove
Nichols but also to the larger history of nineteenth-century sexuality
in the United States. An investigation of Graham came to dominate my
research as I realized that he was the first writer to articulate fully the
physiological principles and anxieties generally associated with the Victorian age. Dr. and Mrs. Nichols became relegated to a single chapter,
and Graham emerged as my subject.

One final note: The figure of Sylvester Graham and the movement
he helped define have achieved new and unanticipated salience in the
1970s. When I first began to teach about Graham's ideas ten years ago,
most of my students responded with a mixture of incredulity and amused
disdain: how could people have taken such stuff seriously? But for a
substantial group, at least, that incredulity and amusement has withered
in the last decade—most dramatically in connection with Graham's pro-
nouncements on diet and living habits. These years have witnessed a
resurgence of vegetarianism, organic diet, and "natural" subsistence
regimen. They have seen an even more widespread anxiety that our individual and collective health is being seriously threatened by a variety
of lethal pollutants—invisible chemicals in the food we buy and the air
we breathe, carcinogenic radiation suffusing our bodies, dangerous dependence on drugs, tobacco, and a general pattern of overconsumption.
Sylvester Graham would surely have understood these fears. While it
can be misleading and irresponsible to make too much of apparent
parallels between one age and another, it may help us understand Sylvester Graham at the points where his ideas strike us as most alien if
we can consider those other points where his fears seem most to resemble our own.

NOTES

1. Sidney Ditzion, *Marriage, Morals, and Sex in America: A History of Ideas* (New York, 1953), pp. 322-329.
2. Richard Shryock, "Sylvester Graham and the Popular Health Movement," *Mississippi Valley Historical Review* 18 (1931): 172-183.
3. William B. Walker, "The Health Reform Movement in the United States, 1830-1870," Ph.D. dissertation, Johns Hopkins University, 1955.
4. Gerald Carson, *Cornflake Crusade* (New York and Toronto, 1957), pp. 43-60.
5. Grace Adams and Edward Hutter, *The Mad Forties* (New York, 1942). Adams and Hutter do not deal directly with Graham, but they discuss all the physiological reforms of the 1840s.
6. Siegfried Giedon, *Mechanization Takes Command: A Contribution to Anonymous History* (Oxford and New York, 1948), pp. 201-208; see also pp. 169-201. In isolating "mechanization," however, Giedon ignores its relationship with other sources of social change.
7. Arthur N. Gilbert, "Doctor, Patient, and Onanistic Diseases in the Nineteenth Century," *Journal of the History of Medicine* 30 (1975): 217-234; James C. Whorton, " 'Tempest in a Flesh-Pot': The Formulation of a Physiological Rationale for Vegetarianism," *Journal of the History of Medicine* 32 (1977): 115-139; H. Tristram Englehardt, "The Disease of Masturbation: Values and the Concept of Disease," *Bulletin of the History of Medicine* 48 (1974): 234-248; John R. Betts, "American Medical Thought on Exercise as the Road to Health, 1820-1860," *Journal of the History of Medicine* 45 (1971): 138-152.
8. Joseph F. Kett, *The Formation of the American Medical Profession, 1780-1860* (New Haven, 1968); William G. Rothstein, *American Physicians in the Nineteenth Century: From Sects to Science* (Baltimore, 1972).
9. Yasukichi Yasuba, *Birth Rates of the White Population in the United States, 1800-1860: An Economic Study* (Baltimore, 1962); James R. Potter, "The Growth of Population in America, 1700-1860," in David Glass and D. E. C. Eversley, eds., *Population in History: Essays in Historical Demography* (Chicago, 1965); Daniel Scott Smith, "The Dating of the American Sexual Revolution: Evidence and Interpretation," in Michael Gordon, ed., *The American Family in Social-Historical Perspective* (New York, 1973), pp. 321-335.
10. Ronald G. Walters, *The Antislavery Appeal: American Abolitionism after 1830* (Baltimore, 1976); Lewis Perry, *Radical Abolitionism: Anarchy and the Government of God in Antislavery Thought* (Ithaca, N.Y., 1973); Ronald G. Walters, ed., *Primers for Prudery: Sexual Advice to Victorian America* (Englewood Cliffs, N.J., 1974); see also Ronald G. Walters, *American Reformers, 1815-1860* (New York, 1978), pp. 145-172.
11. Robert David Thomas, *The Man Who Would Be Perfect: John Humphrey Noyes and the Utopian Impulse* (Philadelphia, 1977); Ronald L. Numbers, *Prophetess of Health: A Study of Ellen G. White* (New York, 1974).
12. Paul Faler, "Cultural Aspects of the Industrial Revolution: Lynn, Massachusetts, Shoemakers and Industrial Morality, 1826-1860," *Labor History* 15 (1974): 367-394; Peter Cominos, "Late-Victorian Sexual Respectability and the Social

System," *International Review of Social History* 8 (1963); 18-48, 216-250; Joseph R. Gusfield, *Symbolic Crusade: Status Politics and the Temperance Movement* (Urbana, Ill., 1963); Charles Rosenberg, "Sexuality, Class, and Role in Nineteenth Century America," *American Quarterly* 25 (1973): 131-153; see also Stephen Nissenbaum, "Careful Love: Sylvester Graham and the Emergence of Victorian Sexual Theory in America, 1830-1840" (Ph.D. diss., University of Wisconsin, 1968).

13. G. J. Barker-Benfield, *The Horrors of the Half-Known Life: Male Attitudes toward Women and Sexuality in Nineteenth-Century America* (New York, 1976); John S. Haller, Jr., and Robin M. Haller, *The Physician and Sexuality in Victorian America* (Urbana, Ill., 1974); Nancy Cott, "Passionlessness: An Interpretation of Victorian Sexual Ideology, 1790-1850," *Signs* 4 (1978-79): 219-236; Linda Gordon, *Woman's Body, Woman's Right: A Social History of Birth Control in America* (New York, 1976); Carroll Smith-Rosenberg, "Beauty, the Beast, and the Militant Woman," *American Quarterly* 23 (1971): 562-584; Carroll Smith-Rosenberg, "The Female World of Love and Ritual," *Signs* 1 (1975): 1-29; see also Charles Rosenberg and Carroll Smith-Rosenberg, "The Female Animal: Medical and Biological Views of Women in the Nineteenth Century," *Journal of American History* 59 (1973): 322-356; Daniel Scott Smith, "Family Limitation, Sexual Control, and Domestic Feminism in Victorian America," in Mary Hartman and Lois Banner, eds., *Clio's Consciousness Raised: New Perspectives on the History of Women* (New York, 1974), pp. 119-136; and Howard Gadlin, "Private Lives and Public Order: A Critical View of Intimate Relations in the United States," in George Levinger and Harold Rausch, eds., *Close Relationships: Perspectives on the Meaning of Intimacy* (Amherst, Mass., 1977), pp. 33-72.

ACKNOWLEDGMENTS

I first became interested in Jacksonian sexuality while serving as research assistant to my graduate advisor, William R. Taylor, then at the University of Wisconsin. He taught me how to think about history, and I regret only that it has taken me so long to acknowledge publicly my gratitude. I received generous fellowships to help me revise the manuscript from the National Endowment for the Humanities and from the Charles Warren Center for Studies in American History at Harvard University, and a Faculty Research Grant for the same purpose from the Graduate School of the University of Massachusetts. But for the effort and encouragement of John C. Burnham, the manuscript probably would not have been published. Critical support (in one or another sense of the phrase) came at various stages from Charles Bowden and Stanley N. Katz at the University of Wisconsin; Douglas Riach at the Charles Warren Center; and Bruce Laurie at the University of Massachusetts.

Norman O. Brown, Bob Gross, and Ronald Walters made helpful comments about specific parts of the manuscript. Christopher Clark discovered and showed me an unpublished letter written by Graham at the end of his life. Peter Knights advised me on how to use the Boston property valuations. Al DeSimone helped me to bring the notes up to date historiographically. Candace Hall assisted me at the Massachusetts Bureau of Vital Records. Sally Ives typed the manuscript with efficiency, understanding, and grace. Paul Boyer and Jack Wilson were always there.

Judy Nissenbaum has seen too much unpleasantness from all this, but I offer it to her with love.

SEX, DIET, AND DEBILITY IN JACKSONIAN AMERICA

1. SYLVESTER GRAHAM AND THE PHYSIOLOGY OF SUBSISTENCE

Ralph Waldo Emerson called him "the prophet of bran bread and pumpkins." In his own day he was widely regarded as a wild-eyed fanatic and a crank, and even many of his own supporters viewed him with a curious mixture of idolatry and exasperation. Like the radical abolitionist William Lloyd Garrison, he became the target of mob violence during the 1830s. Like Garrison, too, he looked for posterity to redeem his reputation. But posterity failed to do so. Sylvester Graham wished to purge the souls of his generation by cleansing their debauched bodies. In his view, the source of the nation's woes lay not in slavery but in diet. In retrospect, his crusade came to appear more trivial than dangerous, and it may be difficult to understand the intensity of his commitment as anything more than the expression of personal gullibility or neurosis. No statue in his memory is to be found alongside that of Garrison on the Boston Common—or anywhere else. His house in Northampton, Massachusetts, which he predicted would become a national shrine, still stands, unmarked and unrecognized, for many years the site of a local tavern. His name is memorialized, devoid of personal associations, only in his one enduring legacy: Graham crackers.

Sylvester Graham may be remembered in that single phrase, but the commercial product to which it refers bears only the most distant and ironic connection to a man who spent most of his adult life in a crusade against just such products. Graham began his career as a temperance worker in the early days of the organized temperance movement. As a result of his work, he became the first important American exponent of vegetarianism and diet reform. His vegetarian ideas were first clearly articulated in a controversial lecture he delivered about the dangers of masturbation and marital excess—the first important expression of a new fear of human sexuality that would become one of the trademarks of the later nineteenth century. Graham himself may have been largely forgotten, but his ideas on these subjects came to find widespread acceptance among middleclass Americans. They were adopted, directly and virtually intact, by the Seventh-Day Adventists; and on a more secular level, they ultimately led to the rise of the modern American breakfast cereal industry. They reemerged at the turn of the twentieth century in surprising quarters: among a diverse group of spiritualists, British socialists (including George Bernard Shaw and H. G. Wells), and Indian pacifists including Mahatma Ghandi—all of whom associated abstinence from animal food with sexual continence.

For Graham himself, the need for vegetable diet and controlled sexuality was based on a coherent and complicated theory of human physiology, a theory that emphasized the lethal dangers of physical stimulation, and hypothesized the existence of a complex network of physiological interconnections that made the human body an exceedingly fragile and vulnerable organism exposed to constant assaults from the outside world.

In retrospect, it was clearly no accident that this theory first emerged in the 1830s. As historians have come to see, these were years of profound change in the way many Americans were living and working. Above all, the Jacksonian period was a time when the marketplace was beginning to replace the household and the community as the major locus of economic activity and social relationships. Set off by the widespread dispersal of the population after 1800 and the subsequent development of new modes of transport, the emergence of a marketplace economy broke up families at the same time it linked distant communities into a single interdependent network. More people were starting to buy rather than to make what they used, and to sell rather than use what they made. These transactions were taking place within an increasingly impersonal setting—a system in which even the most basic products (furniture, clothing, and food) might be produced by people who lived hundreds of miles from the homes in which they were finally used.

As late as 1800, 85 percent of America's manufactured goods were produced in the household, and the bulk of these goods was consumed either by the family that made them or by a neighboring household in the same community. But by the 1830s, this figure had been reduced dramatically. For many people, within a single generation, the household had ceased to be the basic unit of production.

It was to these people that Graham spoke. Nor was it fortuitious that many of them came to associate him almost exclusively with a single point in his general message: the proper preparation of bread. Through the ages, bread had been the basic stuff of human existence—the "staff of life." For ages, too, breadmaking had played a central role in the system of household production—baked on the domestic hearth, from home-grown grain. Yet during these very years, bread itself was becoming just another commercial commodity. The staff of life was removed gradually from household production and coming to be manufactured, marketed, and consumed in the new depersonalized marketplace. By focussing on this change—for all the ridicule it evoked from Emerson and other skeptics— Graham touched a resonant note in the experience of Americans. From this perspective "Graham bread" was a serious, if symbolic, attempt to come to terms with life in a marketplace society; and, if only because this bread has so completely defined Sylvester Graham's place in history, it is a good place to begin an exploration of his ideas.

"In cities and large towns," Graham wrote in 1837, "most people depend on public bakers for their bread." The evidence bears out his statement. In Boston alone, the 1846 city directory listed forty-eight commercial bakeries. Moreover, the bread sold by those bakers was generally manufactured from wheat grown in the distant Ohio Valley. This wheat was less expensive than the New England product because of the greater fertility of midwestern soil and the existence of a network of recently constructed canals that greatly reduced the cost of transportation over great distances. Even in the more fertile agricultural districts of New England such as the Connecticut River Valley, where Sylvester Graham had been born and where he lived after 1838, many people (including farmers) were buying cheaper western flour by the 1830s. Throughout the Northeast, in fact, people were making or purchasing their bread from market flour, raised in distant regions by commercial farmers who remained forever faceless and anonymous to them.[1]

The commercialization of grain agriculture was not simply an abstract development. It had palpable effects on the final product—and Sylvester Graham and his followers may be forgiven if they exaggerated the impact of those effects. Raising wheat for sale in a highly competitive market, commercial farmers were understandably interested in maximizing their production. As Graham noted, such farmers were eager to "extort" from their acreage "the greatest amount of produce, with the least expense of tillage, and with little or no regard to the quality of that produce." In order to "extort" as much as they could from the soil, for example, many commercial farmers by the 1820s were coming to abandon a long-standing reluctance to fertilize their land with animal manures. Graham worried that fertilization, which he considered "unnatural," destroyed the "virgin purity" of "undepraved soil," and that manured soil was "exhausted by [constant] tillage, and debauched by the means which man uses to enrich and stimulate it."[2] The idea that the earth itself could be "debauched" and "exhausted," and that such a process was the result of artificial "stimulation," had its origin in the complex theory of physiology that Graham had developed by the 1830s. The language itself, with its conscious sexual connotations, was characteristic of Graham (as it was of other Jacksonian reformers).

The farmers who cultivated the grain were not the only people responsible for the poor state of store-bought bread. Even more serious offenders were the commercial bakers who prepared and sold it. These men, too, were interested simply in their profit. "Public bakers," Graham wrote, "like other men who serve the public more for the sake of securing their own emolument than for the public good," will inevitably be tempted to resort to whatever "expedients" may promise "to increase the lucrativeness of their business." As Graham pointed out, the quality and price of commercial flour was "very unstable," since it fluctuated wildly in response to changing domestic and foreign markets. For this reason, and in order "to make the most profitable use of such flour as the market affords them," commercial bakers were only too willing to adulterate their already inferior flour with a variety of artificial "chemical agents." These additives, Graham claimed, were known to include "alum, sulphate of zinc, sub-carbonate of magnesia, [and] sulphate of copper." To make matters even worse, many bakers had been able to "disguise their adulterations" by adding such materials as "chalk, pipe clay and plaster of Paris," which served to "increase the weight and whiteness of their bread" without risk of "being detected by the consumers."[3]

But even when commercial bakers refrained from engaging in such shady practices, the bread they sold was still an inferior product. Frequently, it was leavened with the same commercial brewer's yeast that was used in the manufacture of alcoholic beverages. Furthermore (and this is the point to which the name of Sylvester Graham would become irretrievably linked), such bread was baked from "superfine flour"—bolted flour from which the husks of the grain had been removed, and which had been ground up or "refined" to the point where its natural granular texture had been "torture[d] " into an unnatural state of "concentration." In other words, public bakers were vending an early variety of *white bread*, bread with a thin crust and a soft interior that could be prepared more efficiently than the traditional crusty whole wheat product. What soon came to be termed "Graham bread" was in fact nothing more than traditional homegrown and homemade whole wheat bread with a few added twists in preparation and an aggressively ideological rationale.[4]

In his *Treatise on Bread and Bread-Making,* Graham was explicit about this point. Even the most honest of commercial bakers, he insisted, ended up with a product that was invariably inferior to the bread made from "what is called good 'family flour.' " The best bread was always that produced "within the precincts of our own threshholds." There was a "natural sweetness and richness" in such bread that made it "always desirable." It was this, and this only, that could truly be regarded as the staff of life, and Graham wrote almost ecstatically about the few households in which he had stayed during his travels where it had been served to him. But he ruefully acknowledged that such households were few and far between, and that the very possibility of being able to prepare this delicious and wholesome bread had become slim. In an implicit concession to the fact that he was addressing a public that no longer had the means to grow its own flour, Graham urged his audience to purchase the best flour they could find, to grind it themselves with "a modern patent hand-mill," and, of course, to bake it in their own ovens.[5] If Graham bread was a version of traditional bread, it was a version that had come to at least minimal terms with the realities of a marketplace society. Its appeal to tradition was, on a practical level, more symbolic than real. It represented the moral equivalent of vanishing economic self-sufficiency.

Perhaps for this very reason, Graham's analysis of the decline of traditional breadmaking conveyed a moral urgency that transcended the physiological and scientific terms in which it was couched. To Graham, the technological changes that accompanied the transformation of domestic bread into a cheap and potentially lethal article of commerce were a single manifestation of the basic social change that comprised the larger transformation of America in the first third of the nineteenth century.

The ultimate problem with commercial bread was not technological but spiritual. Even though it was extremely helpful to follow carefully

all the "correct rules" of making bread (and there are eighteen pages
devoted to these rules in his *Treatise on Bread-Making*), Graham went
out of his way to argue that the finished product would always be inferior when it was a commercial baker who followed those rules. Precisely because he was a man of commerce, the public baker necessarily
lacked the one crucial element that made for really healthful bread: not
technical know-how, but a "moral sensibility" that comprehends "the
importance of the quality of bread, in relation to the happiness and welfare of those who consume it. "Such a moral sensibility, Graham insisted,
was not to be found in commercial bakers.[6] These men baked their bread
in the impersonal ovens of the marketplace and not on the warm hearth of
the domestic circle. For them, the only effective leaven was cash.

Where was the requisite sensibility to be found? "Who then shall make
our bread?" Graham asked. The answer was obvious:

> It is the wife, the mother only—she who loves her husband and
> her children as woman ought to love, and who rightly perceives
> the relation between the dietetic habits and physical and moral
> conditions of her loved ones, and justly appreciates the importance
> of good bread to their physical and moral welfare,—she alone it is,
> who will be ever inspired by that cordial and unremitting affection
> and solicitude which will excite the vigilance, secure the attention,
> and prompt the action requisite to success, and essential to the
> attainment of that maturity of judgment and skillfulness of opera-
> tion, which are the indispensable attributes of a perfect bread-
> maker.[7]

It was thus an essentially social vision that was evoked in Graham's
mind by the image of well-baked bread: the vision of a domestic idyll,
of a mother nursing her family with bread and affection. It was a historical
vision as well—the sentimentalized memory of a precapitalist order in
which the household functioned simultaneously as a productive unit and
a protective one, where people did not have to rely on the unfeeling ex-
changes of the marketplace for either their physical or their emotional
sustenance. Graham recognized and lamented the fact that such a world
had all but disappeared. In a highly significant and uncharacteristically
lyrical passage, the ordinarily strident reformer explicitly associated the
twilight of that world with the time of his own childhood and the childhood of his generation at the turn of the nineteenth century:

Who that can look back 30 or 40 years to those blessed days of
New England's prosperity and happiness, when our good mothers
used to make the family bread, but can well remember how long
and how patiently those excellent matrons stood over their bread
troughs, kneading and molding their dough? And who with such
recollections cannot also well remember the delicious bread that
those mothers used invariably to set before them? There was a
natural sweetness and richness in it which made it always desirable;
and which we cannot now vividly recollect, without feeling a strong
desire to partake again of such bread as our mothers used to make
for us in the days of our childhood.[8]

Graham himself had good reason to sentimentalize this nurturing social
environment, and to shun the impersonal and menacing capitalist marketplace that had replaced it. His own family had once been a prominent
and stable part of its community—for fifty years his father had served as
its minister—but in the course of his childhood Graham was the witness
and victim of his family's total disintegration as a coherent institutional
unit. The "blessed days of New England's prosperity and happiness" had
come to a rude end with the death of his father, the emotional collapse
of his mother, and the failure of anyone else effectively to replace them.
Sylvester Graham's paternal grandfather, the Reverend John Graham,
was a Scotsman—a minister and a 1714 graduate of the University of
Glasgow—who had emigrated to the New World four years after his
graduation. He occupied several pulpits in the western part of New England, and it was there that his first son and Sylvester's father, John
Graham, Jr., was born in 1722. The younger John Graham was graduated
from Yale College in 1740 and licensed to preach the following year, just
as the first important religious revival in America, the Great Awakening,
was sweeping through New England. Both father and son were fervent
supporters of the awakening. In 1746, twenty-four-year-old John Graham,
Jr.was ordained as pastor of a new congregation (spawned by a combination of religious upheaval and population growth) in West Suffield, a
small town in the Connecticut River Valley just south of the Massachusetts
border. He retained this pulpit, and the prominent position in his community that went with it, for exactly half a century until his death in
1796, at the age of seventy-four. During these years he married twice,
and his two wives bore him a total of seventeen children, all of whom
survived their father. Sylvester Graham was the last of these seventeen

children. When he was born, in 1794, his father was seventy-two years old and had less than two years to live.[9]

Ruth Graham, the minister's second wife and Sylvester's mother, was only forty-one when her elderly husband died. It was her job to rear the seven children she had borne, all of whom were still young enough to be living at home. But, since John Graham had died without leaving a will, she was left without any clear holdings in his 1000-pound estate. (John Graham's ten children by his first wife had all moved away by this time, and most of them apparently had received property settlements while he was still alive.) It was not until 1800—four years after his death—that a distribution of the estate finally was made. But by that time other difficulties had emerged within the Graham family. Ruth Graham failed to remarry, and she seems to have become emotionally unable to care adequately for her children. As Sylvester Graham later said, "My mother's health sunk under her complicated trials, the family was broken up, and . . . I fell into the hands of strangers." When Sylvester was three years old, he was sent to live with neighbors—a fairly common practice in late eighteenth-century rural communities. Two years later he was lodged with a local tavernkeeper, but after falling seriously ill, he moved into the household of one of his married half sisters. In 1801, when he was six, in a sad contrast to his later recollection of the times "when our good mothers used to make the family bread," the county probate court decreed that Ruth Graham was "in a deranged state of mind," and the selectmen of West Suffield appointed a local farmer to be his legal guardian.[10]

This arrangement lasted for five years, during which young Sylvester worked as a "farmer's boy." When he was eleven, one of his older brothers sent him to school in distant New York City, but the unfamiliar life there made him unhappy, and at his own request he soon returned to West Suffield. For a time during his mid-teens Sylvester again lived with his mother, finding employment where he was able. At one point he worked briefly in a local paper mill, but after a month he quit and moved in with still another local farmer. Ever dissatisfied, he left the farm and worked at different times as assistant to a travelling horse dealer and as a clerk in various shops in the area. Falling ill at age sixteen, he was sent to live with one of his sisters in Middlebury, Vermont. At nineteen, in an effort to become a schoolteacher, he spent some four months studying with a private tutor, but after teaching in several small towns for a short time, exhaustion and illness forced him to abandon this occupation. In a state of intense depression he moved to Albany to stay with another of his sisters, and then in 1817, at age twenty-three, to Newark, New Jersey, the home of still another sibling.[11]

It was sometime during these years that Graham for the first time began to emerge from his long miasma. As a teenager, he had been ardently fond of attending social gatherings—especially parties and balls. While he never drank the hard liquor served at these affairs, his abstinence stemmed from physical distaste rather than any principled objection. Nevertheless, as he later recalled, the pressure of his peers, and his concern for their good opinion of him had exposed him to "many temptations" along these lines—temptations that were especially intense because, as he pointedly recalled, "I had no particular employment, and was left almost entirely to follow my own will." On one of these occasions, though, he finally discovered the true direction and force of his will, and in the process the vocation that had so long eluded him.[12]

The crucial event was what Graham later referred to as "one of those peculiar trials which young men too seldom have the courage to endure." A group of friends had invited him to a party at a local tavern. Graham agreed to attend, but because it embarrassed him to be the only nondrinker in the group, he proposed that no alcohol be served at the affair. His stipulation was ostensibly accepted all around, and the party got under way in pleasant fashion. But, Graham unwittingly had been set up by his friends. Late in the evening one of them called for a glass of "rum-sling." Immediately a hush fell over the gorup, and "all eyes were turned" on Graham to see how he would react to the challenge. He protested, but his protests were rebuffed. When the glass, by now emptied and refilled several times, was finally handed to Graham, he tried to pass it along without raising it to his lips. That was what the assembly had been waiting for, and they taunted him: " 'He is too stingy to call for his glass and that is the reason he won't drink!' " It was, as Graham later acknowledged, "a most trying moment." The idea of being thought stingy by his friends was "almost intolerable." But while Graham "felt the reproach keenly," he was "determined not to yield." He pretended to ignore the barrage of taunts, until finally, when the humiliation seemed complete, the young man sitting next to Graham drank the glass of rum.

It was at this point that Graham acted to prove he was not stingy, to regain his dignity—and to assume control of the situation. As soon as his glass had been drained, Graham dramatically ordered the tavernkeeper to bring another glass of rum—*for him.* When the fresh drink arrived, Graham "planted it with firmness in the middle of the table," rose out of his chair, and with a "stern voice" announced to the rest of the party, "gentlemen, good night." Now it was his friends' turn to feel embarrassed. They attempted to detain Graham, but, ignoring their pleas just as they had previously ignored his protests, Graham calmly picked up his hat and walked out of the tavern. The spirit had gone out of the joke, and the group soon dispersed. In retrospect, Graham felt this was a moment of profound significance for him. Not only had he saved his friends from a probable "debauch," but—of even greater importance—the incident "gave a direction to the whole course of my life."

Despite Graham's retrospective comment that few young men would have had the "courage to endure" such a "trial," the episode was similar in form to the experience of many directionless young men who came of age in the Jacksonian years, involving as it did Graham's loss of shame and dependence and his simultaneous discovery of a new sense of personal autonomy and power. In characteristically Jacksonian fashion, too, the incident at the tavern moved Graham away from his purely personal and somewhat abashed reluctance to drink and into what he called an "open and frequent" effort to persuade others to believe and act as he did. Graham began to "contend" passionately with his fellow farmhands about the evils of drink. Then, early in 1823, he delivered his first public lecture on the subject to a debating society near his hometown of West Suffield, Connecticut, and shortly afterwards he organized an informal temperance club there.

Later the same year, at the age of twenty-nine, Graham entered Amherst Academy (a preparatory school associated with the fledgling Amherst College) in order to prepare for the evangelical ministry. But he was unable to adjust to the academic routine. After a short stay at the academy he fell into a state of "mental despondency and wretchedness," and before the end of his first semester, he was dismissed from the institution, apparently on a trumped-up charge of assault. His dismissal, coming on top of his already depressed state, soon led to an acute physical and emotional collapse. In this condition, he made his way (for reasons that remain obscure) to the Rhode Island coastal town of Little Compton. There he was slowly nursed back to health by the two daughters of a sea captain at whose house he was staying. In September 1824, Graham was married to the older of these two women.[13]

With his health restored, and a wife to support, Graham now resumed his preparation for the ministry. Probably because his attempt to gain a more formal education had failed, he resorted to the increasingly dated practice of studying privately with the local parish minister—in this case the very man who had officiated at his wedding in Little Compton. In 1826 Graham was licensed to preach; and after his ordination as an evangelist two years later, he moved back to the Newark area where his mother, confined to an institution, was still living.[14] At the age of thirty-four, Sylvester Graham finally seemed embarked on a career—the same ministerial career as his father and grandfather before him.

But, unlike his clerical forebears, Graham never managed to settle down with a parish of his own, and within two years he had abandoned the ministry altogether. He served for a while as guest preacher in the New Jersey community of Belvedere, and for more than a year during 1829 and 1830, he served as acting minister to a small congregation in the nearby town of Bound Brook. (There, as an account book reveals, his wife baked bread from locally grown flour.) But a large part of Graham's new congregation turned against him when he delivered a series of sermons against intemperance. Even though his admonitions resulted in the closing of a nearby distillery and the formation of a local temperance society, Graham's position in the Bound Brook community had become tenuous. Under the circumstances, he was quick to accept the next job that was offered. In June 1830, Sylvester Graham became an agent of the Pennsylvania Temperance Society.[15]

Graham immediately moved to Philadelphia, and in his new capacity as temperance reformer he travelled around eastern Pennsylvania, lecturing in churches and factories and helping to form new local and county temperance societies. In this capacity Graham seems to have been notably successful—his lively and impassioned style of extemporaneous speaking began to attract large audiences—and by early 1831, he was asked to deliver a series of lectures on the subject in New York City. He did so that summer and again the ensuing autumn (at which time he was prevailed on to repeat his entire series several times). At this point Graham had come to consider himself not simply a temperance reformer, but a lecturer on a far more inclusive subject that he called "The Science of Human Life," and over the next few years he would come to expand his repertoire to cover the cholera epidemic (which ravaged the United States in 1832), the importance of sexual chastity and vegetarian diet, and, of course, the virtues of bran bread. For the rest of the decade he delivered these lectures through-out the Atlantic states and New England, and eventually he travelled as far afield as upstate New York. His lectures on cholera, sexuality, and bread-making were published between 1832 and 1837 (each of them going through a number of editions), and in 1839 he published his magnum opus, *Lectures on the Science of Human Life,* in two volumes of more than 1,200 pages.[16]

But the growing celebrity of his ideas, along with his contentious and abrasive manner, made Graham a controversial figure. As one of his sup-porters later recalled in an obituary notice, Graham was a gifted orator, but his temperament was married by "combativeness, extreme cautiousness, excessive ideality, and more than full self-esteem."[17] He was publicly mobbed at least three times, once in Portland, Maine, in 1834 and twice in Boston during the winter of 1837. The first time an angry crowd prevented him from delivering his lecture on chastity to an all female audience, and the second time he was attacked by a group of commercial butchers and bakers who feared his ideas were bad for their business.

Graham's eventual eclipse may have been hastened by the fact that he came to be dismissed as a charlatan by several respectable medical publica-tions (notably the *Boston Medical and Surgical Journal*) which had initially welcomed his work as a serious contribution to the field of personal health.[18] Furthermore, like William Lloyd Garrison (who had likewise been mobbed in Boston during the mid-1830s, and who had similarly been dismissed as a fanatic by the more moderate members of his own party), Graham often personally alienated even those followers who were ideologically close to him. He also remained aloof from the very people who paid him the homage he craved. He never stayed in any of the "Graham boardinghouses" opened by his disciples in Boston and New York during the mid-1830s in an attempt to institutionalize healthy diet and regimen. He maintained only minimal contact with the American Physiological Society, a Boston group he helped to found in 1837. He took no part in editing the *Graham Journal of Health and Longevity,* published from 1837 to 1839 by his disciple, David Cam-bell, who also managed the Graham boardinghouse in Boston. (Graham once acknowledged privately that he tended to act with "gall and vinegar" toward the very people for whom he most deeply cared.)

In the last decade of his life, Sylvester Graham was effectively cut off from the intellectual and institutional currents he had helped set in motion. After 1839 he gave up his itinerant lecturing and settled down into semi-retirement with his wife and two children in Northampton, Massachusetts, just twenty-five miles upriver from the town in which he had been born. There he spent the last dozen years of his life, something of a crotchety local character, writing self-pitying poetry, letters to the editor of the local newspaper, and a lengthy defense of vegetarian diet on biblical grounds. He died in 1851, after violating his own strictures by taking liquor and meat in a last desperate attempt to recover his health.[19]

It would be naive to attribute Sylvester Graham's chronic career problems simply to the disruptions he experienced in his early life. After all, the years in which Graham was coming of age was a time when such newly emerging careers as those of professional lecturer and writer were not yet able to provide a reliable source of income. Nevertheless, the failure of Graham's family to ease his way into adulthood certainly played an important role in determining the difficult course of his later life. In any case, this particular failure mirrored the larger transformation of American rural society in the early years of the nineteenth century.

The disintegration of traditional kinship ties in this period is dramatically revealed in the contrast between the two different "families" that Sylvester Graham's father sired and reared over his long career: The ten children of his first marriage, born between 1749 and 1768, and the seven children of his second marriage, born between 1780 and 1792. Of the six sons and four daughters born to John Graham's first wife, each of the four daughters married, and married well; and five of the six sons attained some degree of prosperity.

John Graham's eldest son was sent, like his father before him, to Yale College. By graduation he had become interested in medicine, and went directly from Yale to earn a medical degree from King's College (Columbia) in New York City. He established his practice with the professional assistance of one of his father's brothers, a prominent physician who lived outside New York City in suburban White Plains. Largely because of these advantages, all of them derived from the concern and connections of his family, the eldest son was able to establish an extremely successful practice of his own. It was only appropriate, and no doubt entirely expected of him, that some twenty years later he trained and supported one of *his* younger brothers—the last son born of John Graham's first marriage—and helped him to complete his medical studies in London and Edinburgh. A third son, who as a young man received his start in the form of a generous gift of real estate from his father, became a well-to-do land speculator and merchant in western New York after the Revolutionary War. Another son became a prosperous if somewhat shady merchant in the Boston area; and the last a wealthy land speculator in South Carolina.[20]

It is significant that the children whom John Graham fathered by his first marriage were all established in their careers well before their father died. (They ranged in age from twenty-eight to forty-seven at the time of his death.) Because a dozen years elapsed between the birth of the last child of his first marriage and the first child of his second, the oldest of the seven children of this second marriage was only sixteen when the father died, and the youngest—Sylvester—was not quite two. All the children of the first marriage, moreover, had left the West Suffield area by this time, and it appears that the two "families" did not have any contact after the father's death. Since Sylvester Graham's mother herself never remarried—indeed, since she was declared insane after seven years of widowhood—it is clear that what remained of the Graham family in West Suffield after 1796 had no other role in the community than as its wards.

There is an obvious difference between the careers of the seven children of John Graham's second marriage and the ten children of his first. Two of the four girls born of this second union never married, and a third remained single until she was nearly forty. The most stable of the seven children, both economically and (from what can be inferred) emotionally, were the two oldest, both boys. (They were also the only ones to have reached adolescence at the time of their father's death.) Even these two children enjoyed only modest success. One of them, Isaac King Graham, remained in West Suffield almost until his death; all that is known of him is that he was quiet and attended church regularly. The other, Charles Graham, began his career as an accountant in New York City. He later moved to Newark, where he made a good marriage and ended his days in comfortable circumstances as a cashier in a banking house.

It was Charles Graham who tried to keep what Sylvester would later term the "little remnant" of the Graham family together. When Charles moved to Newark in 1817 he was followed by his mother, three of his four sisters, and his twenty-three-year-old brother Sylvester. Whatever aid Charles Graham did provide, however, was too little and too late to guide his sisters into marriage or his younger brother into a career. All he was able to offer was a modicum of respite from the burden of living in a community where the name of Graham had once carried an assurance of stability, prosperity, and respect.

Sylvester Graham came to maturity, then, without much effective help or guidance from his family or his community. When at length he discovered his vocation, he did so substantially on his own—and then only when he was in his mid-thirties, after a long series of false starts accompanied by chronic bouts of debilitating illness and depression. The career in which he finally achieved some measure of success was one that represented the essence of the emerging world of the capitalist marketplace. Like his better remembered cohort, Ralph Waldo Emerson (and at almost exactly the same time), Graham first entered the established ministry but soon abandoned it in order to become a professional writer and travelling lecturer, forced to deal with an ever-changing array of impersonal and undependable audiences.

It is, therefore, a revealing irony that Sylvester Graham tried to romanticize the secure family life he had never known. As he grew older he developed an interest in his genealogy, especially in what he insisted were the Graham clan's royal origins in Scotland. In his last years he openly lamented the way the family had disintegrated over the years. In two poignant letters written late in life to his brother Isaac, who was still living in West Suffield, and whom he had apparently not seen in some time—"I trust you are living, for if you were not the newspapers at least would inform me of your death"—Sylvester Graham pleaded for "a measure of cordial love and harmony between the little remnant of our father's family." Referring to the two of his sisters who were still alive, he admitted that "Jerusha's alienation from me I fear will never be overcome—and now Harriet is also torn from me I fear by the demoniacal infatuation of one of her children." He added desperately, addressing his brother in biblical language, " 'Wilt thou also go away?' " He reminded Isaac that "when I was a little, unprotected fatherless boy, you were not only a brother but in a father's stead to me"; and speaking of the father he could scarcely have remembered, he asked, "Could our venerated Sire return to earth . . . would he not say to us—'My little children love one another?'"[21]

It is characteristic of both his personal and his professional life, that what Graham seems to have craved most of all was the feeling of being remembered and cared for, and that what he most feared was the possibility of being forgotten or ignored. He exhibited no desire

that his family be knit together by any bonds other than those of
mutual concern. All he wanted was for his family to be a community of
feeling. He did not expect it to provide any services other than emotional
ones. Within this emotional community he saw his own role as wholly
passive—much like that of the children he remembered, feeding on "the
delicious bread [their] mothers used unvariably to set before them,"
watching their mothers stand "long and patiently . . . over their bread
troughs, kneading and molding their dough" in a manner appropriate
to those who love their families "as woman ought to love." (The loveliness of this scene, as Graham described it, lay both in the security, love,
and nourishment the mother lavished on her family, and in the passivity,
the absence of reciprocal responsibility, with which they received it. There
may be some significance in the fact that Graham married a woman who
literally was his nurse.)

Graham's sentimentalization of a protective family life he had never
known finds its direct parallel in the way he extolled the superiority
of a personalized, self-sufficient society even as he travelled around the
lecture circuit addressing faceless urban audiences he rarely encountered
more than a few times. Each of these paradoxical stances expressed perfectly the complex dynamics of Jacksonian social change: they provided
a means by which both Graham and his disciples were able to begin making the difficult psychological transition into a capitalist society. Graham
was not the only member of his generation to idealize the remembered
past at the very point when that past had ceased to wield significant force
in the life of the present. All over Western society, both in America and
in Europe, nineteenth-century reformers, writers, and painters were creating nostalgic pictures of yeomen with their hoes, shepherds attending to
their flocks, and patient women at their spinning wheels (or, in Graham's
case, at their ovens). The toil and monotony of these tasks were forgotten
as they were transformed by the light of nostalgia into scenes of beauty
and harmony. By the very act of looking back, the emergent bourgeoisie
was able to come to terms with the future.

When Sylvester Graham romanticized the life of the traditional household, he unknowingly helped prepare women to find a new role as the
guardians of domestic virtue, just as he helped prepare men—himself included—to adjust to the demands of the capitalist marketplace. The passive security Graham associated with the image of protective mothers
preparing bread for their beloved children was as much a vestige of the

past as was wholesome family flour. The present-day order had no room either for domestic bread or for the trusting security it symbolized. The world of Jacksonian America was everywhere fraught with menace. Commerical bakers, with their undetectably adulterated flour and their dismaying lack of "Moral sensibility," were only the tip of the iceberg. In every area of modern life people were faced with similar situations— distant farmers who could not be trusted because they could not be known, or unscrupulous merchants who could not be trusted because they were more concerned with turning a profit than with securing the well-being of those who were forced to depend on them. American society, Graham worried, was being consumed by its "untiring pursuit of wealth." At each turn, people were besieged "every luxury . . . that the market can supply."[22]

Commercially baked bread was only a metaphor of the Jacksonian marketplace itself—a place of fevered chaos, laden with products manufactured by invisible men and corrupted with invisible poisons. Anonymity encouraged conspiracy; consumers were beset at every point by forces that threatened their well-being and even their survival. In the face of such a minatory situation, old fashioned passivity and trust were a potentially lethal indulgence. It was necessary to be wary and alert, on constant guard.

Sylvester Graham shared this phobic vision of Jacksonian society with many other Americans of his day. Anti-Masons focussed on the Masonic order as the source of the threat, nativists attributed it to the increasing influx of immigrants, and abolitionists blamed the slave conspiracy. Andrew Jackson himself pointed the finger of guilt at the "monster" Bank of the United States. In Sylvester Graham's particular version, the threat primarily was physiological in nature—directed against the individual human organism rather than against the body politic. Inverting the process by which traditional political theorists had used "organic" language to describe the social order, Graham applied the rhetoric of late eighteenth-century republican social philosophy to the individual human organism. The human body, he claimed, had its own proper form of "government," based on a natural "constitution" which in turn provided for "constitutionally established laws." This physiological government was "endowed" with certain specific "powers," and when these powers were misused or undermined, the inevitable consequence was a state of "anarchical depravity" or "despotism." [23]

Graham was able to describe in detail the precise nature of the physiological "constitution" and its extraordinary vulnerability to the hostile
elements constantly threatening its annihilation—disease, diet, and sexuality. Graham had prepared himself to deal with these subjects in purely
scientific terms. He prided himself on the depth of his technical competence. He allowed himself to be addressed as "Dr. Graham" even though
he had received no medical training. He had, however, read in limited
areas of recent physiological theory. It was from some key ideas he gained
in his reading, along with several predispositions he picked up from his
work in the temperance movement, that Graham developed the complex
and coherent body of principles he proudly dubbed, as early as 1830,
"The Science of Human Life." The process by which he came to formulate
these principles is the subject of this book.

Graham derived two of his key ideas from the work of a pair of French
medical theorists, Xavier Bichat (1771-1802) and François Broussais (1772-
1838). Bichat had proposed that all living organisms were engaged in a
continuous struggle for survival against the inorganic forces that surrounded
them: life itself was a constant battle between the principles of vitality and
those of physics and chemistry, and death was simply the victory of the
latter over the former. Broussais, another French theorist, had proposed
that food and drink, upon which living organisms depended for their survival but which literally invaded them from without, constituted the single
greatest threat to vitality. From Broussais, then, Graham picked up the
idea that it was the digestive system that formed the crucial battleground
in the struggle between organic and inorganic forces.

A third important principle that Graham derived from his reading involved the connection between two bodily conditions: *stimulation* and
debility. Until the end of the eighteenth century, these two states were
universally conceived to be opposite and mutually exclusive. Debility (that
is, weakness or lack of vital energy) was generally regarded as the more
dangerous of the two states—and artificial stimulation was its obvious
antidote. (For this reason, people who were exhausted from illness or
from hard work generally took stimulants such as alcohol or meat in order
to restore their health and strength.) But late in the eighteenth century,
the Philadelphia physician and statesman, Benjamin Rush, proposed that
artificial stimulation, far from being a cure for debility, was actually its
most common cause. Alcohol and similar stimulants, in Rush's view, served
only to further weaken a person who was in a debilitated state. Rush's

ideas gained widespread acceptance in his native Philadelphia; indeed, they placed an important role in causing that city to become a major center of the emerging temperance movement in the late 1820s.

Graham probably encountered Rush's work, along with that of Bichat and Broussais, about the time he moved to Philadelphia in 1830 to become an agent of the Pennsylvania Temperance Society. By the end of that year, he had begun to integrate these ideas, and others, into the system he called "The Science of Human Life." To the end of his career, Graham tried to convey the impression that the principles he was expounding in his books and lectures were his own personal discoveries, perhaps confirmed but never influenced by his readings in medical literature. This impression was an integral part of his own self-image as a kind of romantic "natural" who was able to perceive the true nature of things precisely because he had not been corrupted by the artifices of modern civilization—artifices that might include formal book-learning.[24]

In a sense Graham was right. In a very real way, he invented these ideas for himself even though he had read them elsewhere, and he did so in a serious and original effort to come to terms with his own experience and that of his generation. If Xavier Bichat defined life as a desperate struggle between organic and inorganic principles, for Graham that definition became a symbol of the struggle of the localized rural world into which he had been born to fend off the powerful incursions of a depersonalized marketplace society. Similarly, if Benjamin Rush postulated that "artificial" stimulation led only to exhaustion and debility, Graham used that idea as a powerful way of portraying the fevered quality of Jacksonian life— and its deleterious effects on those who experienced it.

Graham urged his audience to adopt a mode of living premised on minimal consumption and the systematic effort to achieve inner serenity. "The Science of Human Life" was ultimately Graham's personal attempt, and in its own way a pathetically eloquent one, to provide what might be termed a physiology of subsistence, a practical strategy by which he and his countrymen might survive in alien, unsettling social terrain.

NOTES

1. Sylvester Graham, *Lectures on the Science of Human Life*, 2 vols. (Boston, 1839), 2:423; Boston Directory for 1846 (Boston, 1847), The *New England Inquirer* [Amherst, Mass.], April 3, 1828, contains an advertisement for "85 bbls. Rochester Superfine Flour" (reference courtesy of Christopher Clark). A fine discussion of

economic and social change in the area where Graham was reared, but with wider geographical implications, is Christopher Clark, "The Household Economy, Market Exchange and the Rise of Capitalism in the Connecticut Valley, 1800-1860," 13 *Journal of Social History* (1979): 169-189.

2. Graham, *Science*, 2:418-419. See also Sylvester Graham, *A Treatise on Bread, and Bread-Making* (Boston, 1837), pp. 33-34. (The *Treatise on Bread* was incorporated almost verbatim into the *Lectures on the Science of Human Life.*) Clarence Danhoff, *Change in Agriculture: The Northern United States, 1820-1870* (Cambridge, 1969), pp. 257-262, discusses the increasing use of manures in this period. Graham argued that the odor of manure could be detected in flour milled from wheat grown on fertilized land.

3. Graham, *Science*, 2:424.

4. Ibid., 2:423. Graham maintained (pp. 428-430) that "a due proportion of innutritious matter in our food is as essential to the health and functional integrity of our alimentary organs, as a due proportion of nutritious matter is to the sustenance of our bodies"; in addition, bran was "one of the most soothing substances in nature." Whatever the merits of Graham's argument, the fact is that bread had been prepared from unbolted grain for centuries as a matter of course. "White bread" did not become common in either America or England until the nineteenth century—and even then it was to be found mostly in urban commercial bakeries. See John Burnett, *Plenty and Want: A Social History of Diet in England from 1815 to the Present Day* (London, 1966), pp. 56, 83; J. C. Drummond and Anne Wilbraham, *The Englishman's Food: A history of five centuries of English diet,* rev. ed. (London, 1958), pp. 186-190, 295-299; and Siegfried Giedon, *Mechanization Takes Command: A Contribution to Anonymous History* (New York, 1948), pp. 169-208. In any case, Graham was not even the first American to stress the healthful properties of bran bread. Edward Hitchcock, an Amherst College professor, had recommended much the same recipe in his 1829 book, *Dyspepsy Forestalled* (Northampton, 1831), and a Philadelphia newspaper carried an advertisement for "dyspepsia bread," baked from unbolted wheat flour, at the very time Graham was beginning to lecture on temperance in that city (*Poulson's American Daily Advertiser,* July 20, 1830).

5. Graham, *Science*, 2: 425; *Treatise on Bread,* pp. 39, 49, 131; Giedon, *Mechanization Takes Command,* p. 205.

6. Graham, *Science*, 2:455.

7. Ibid., 2:455-456. See also *Treatise on Bread,* pp. 43-49, 105.

8. Graham, *Science*, 2:448-449.

9. Helen Graham Carpenter, *The Rev. John Graham of Woodbury, Connecticut and His Descendents* (Chicago, 1942), pp. 6-90. The length of John Graham's tenure, the large number of children he sired, and the fact that all of the children survived him, were unusual.

10. Ibid. The autobiographical quotation appeared in William Goodell's magazine, *Genius of Temperance,* May 5, 1831. The inheritance Graham finally received in 1801 amounted to $50.

11. Biographical information from Edith Cole, "Sylvester Graham, Lecturer on

the Science of Human Life: The Rhetoric of a Dietary Reformer" (Ph.D. diss.,
Indiana Univeristy, 1975), pp. 9-12; Mildred Naylor, "Sylvester Graham, 1794-1851,"
Annals of Medical History, series 3, 4 (1941): 236-240; Carpenter, *Rev. John Graham*,
p. 184; and the *Genius of Temperance*, May 5, 1831.

12. Graham recalled this episode in a letter to the *Genius of Temperance*, May 5,
1831.

13. Cole, "Sylvester Graham," p. 16; *Northampton Courier*, July 15, 1840; Naylor,
"Sylvester Graham," pp. 236-237.

14. Carpenter, *Rev. John Graham*, p. 184; Naylor, "Sylvester Graham," p. 237.

15. *Genius of Temperance*, May 25, 1831; Cole, "Sylvester Graham," pp. 15-18;
Naylor, "Sylvester Graham," pp. 236-240. The manuscript records of the Bound
Brook Presbyterian Church do not mention Graham's association with that church,
nor does the manuscript of an address (on deposit with the church records) delivered
by Graham's successor on the twenty-fifth anniversary of his pastorate. Graham is,
however, discussed in a published history of the church: Joseph H. Kler, M.D., *God's
Happy Cluster: 1688-1963, History of the Bound Brook Presbyterian Church* (n.p.,
1963), pp. 64, 73. The only reference to Graham's ordination in 1826 is in the
Reverend Mortimer Blake, *Centennial History of the Mendon Association of Congregational Ministers* (Boston, 1853), pp. 78, 309.

16. *Genius of Temperance*, March 30, 1831, April 6, 1831, and June 1, 1831;
Pennsylvania Temperance Society, *Annual Report of the Managers of the Pennsylvania
Society for Discouraging the Use of Ardent Spirits* (Philadelphia, 1831), p. 22;
Othniel A. Pendleton, Jr., "The Influence of the Evangelical Churches upon Humani-
tarian Reform: A Case Study Giving Particular Attention to Philadelphia, 1790-
1840," *Journal of the Presbyterian Historical Society* 25 (1947): 22; Cole, "Sylvester
Graham," pp. 20-22, 65-69.

17. Russell T. Trall, "Biographical Sketch of Sylvester Graham," *Water-Cure Journal* 12 (1851): 110. (Trall's terminology is phrenological—the relationship among
Grahamism, phrenology, and the water-cure, and Trall's association with these movements, is discussed here in Chapter 9.) Another interesting reference to Graham's abrasive temperament can be found in Theodore Dwight Weld's notation on a letter he
received from Graham, in Gilbert H. Barnes and Dwight L. Dumond, eds., *Letters of
Theodore Dwight Weld, Angelina Grimké Weld, and Sarah Grimké, 1822-1844*, 2
vols. (New York, 1934), 2:755.

18. Compare, for instance, the favorable review of Graham's *Lecture on Chastity*
that appeared in the *Boston Medical and Surgical Journal* in 1835 with the disdain-
ful materials printed in the same periodical through much of the following year.

19. Trall, "Biographical Sketch," p. 111.

20. This and the following material is gleaned from Carpenter, *Rev. John
Graham*, pp. 123-190.

21. Sylvester Graham to Isaac King Graham, ibid., pp. 188-189. Another letter
written three years later to the same brother consists almost entirely of queries about
the whereabouts and condition of various forgotten members of the family: ibid.,
p. 189. Graham's interest in the family's genealogy is revealed in ibid., pp. 55-56.

22. Graham, *Science*, 2:401.

23. Sylvester Graham, *A Lecture to Young Men, on Chastity, intended also for the serious consideration of parents and guardians* (Providence, 1834), pp. 63, 165-169. This inversion of republican political rhetoric is the origin of such modern usages as referring to walking for one's health as taking a "constitutional."

24. See, for example, *Science*, 1: v-ix. In cultivating this image, Graham was by no means unique: a number of writers who flourished during the Jacksonian period seemed to believe they could enhance their credibility by asserting that they had never read a single book in the area of their competence.

2. THE NEW CHASTITY OF THE 1830s

Sylvester Graham went on the defensive when he published his *Lecture to Young Men on Chastity*. He recognized the risks in writing openly about such a subject, but he insisted that these were mild compared with the danger of remaining quiet. It was the silence of decent men in the face of increasingly open and shameless sexual abuses that had led curious minds to seek information from "mercenary and polluted hands." It was time for well-meaning men of education to speak out and disseminate the facts "as early as the young mind can be made to understand the subject accurately." For this reason Graham decided, early in 1834, to publish the controversial address he had been delivering in different cities for two full years.[1]

It was an address he had not wanted to deliver in the first place. He had been forced into it by a continual stream of "entreaties, and importunities, and heart-touching—and I might truly say heart-rending—appeals" from the young men who had attended his temperance lectures as early as 1830. Only in response to such appeals had Graham reluctantly agreed to speak on this "delicate subject." Even so, his decision to publish came in response to an even more pressing need: the recent publication of a spate of openly immoral books, "extensive, bold, and efficient efforts to encourage illicit and promiscuous commerce between the sexes." Graham named no names, but his list certainly included Robert Dale Owen's *Moral Physiology* (1829) and Charles Knowlton's *Fruits of Philosophy* (1832), the first works on birth control to be printed in the United States. Such books, Graham believed, were taking their toll, for masturbation, fornication, and adultery, and even "sexual excess within the pale of wedlock," were all widespread and increasing "rapidly."[2]

It is difficult to judge the accuracy of Graham's claim. But this much is clear: the early 1830s were a time that witnessed the sudden emergence of an unprecedented public apprehensiveness about human sexuality. It was a new development. As a number of historians have shown, the seventeenth-century Puritans were hardly "puritanical" about sexual matters, and eighteenth-century American society was characterized by an extraordinarily high rate of premarital pregnancy. (Indeed, the latter part of that century may have been sexually the most open period in American history.)[3] When young Benjamin Franklin, for example, composed the famous list of thirteen virtues designed to permit him to attain "moral perfection," he placed *chastity* twelfth on the list, and he gave it an operational definition so hedged with qualifiers as to cramp his style hardly at all: "*Rarely* use venery *but for health or offspring*—never to dulness, weakness, or the injury of your own or another's reputation."[4] Franklin's restrictions notably did not include marriage.

Nor did the eighteenth-century clergy respond to such attitudes and practices by publishing a spate of sermons or other tracts denouncing them. Printed works about sexual misconduct were rare in the colonial period. There was, to be sure, an occasional foray against adultery. Benjamin Wadsworth of Boston's Brattle Street Church published a sermon on the subject in 1716, and almost exactly a century later "Parson" Mason Locke Weems (author of the popular *Life of Washington*) composed a somewhat racier tract along the same lines. But, not a single work appeared on the subject of fornication. In 1723 Wadsworth's Boston colleague, Cotton Mather, anonymously published a short pamphlet that dealt in harsh but vague terms with the evils of masturbation. The following year, in response to Mather's tract and possibly at his behest, there appeared a Boston reprint—the "10th edition," claimed the title page—of an anonymous, more explicit, sixty-five page work entitled *Onania*, which had first appeared in London some ten years earlier.[5] *Onania* had two or three more American editions in the course of the century. As far as I have been able to determine, this list comprises the bibliography of cautionary literature about sex published in America before 1830.

It would be misleading to attribute the scarcity of material to modesty about discussing such matters in public. During the same period there appeared a substantial body of *noncautionary* literature about sexuality. For example, scores of titles were published on the treatment of venereal disease. More important, however, were the "facts-of-life" books, as they would later be known. The most famous and easily the most popular were four anonymous titles that often were published together in a single volume and known collectively as *The Works of Aristotle, the Great Philosopher.* These books were reprinted more than any other medical work in America in the last half of the eighteenth century and the first quarter of the nineteenth. The most widely read of the four, *Aristotle's Master Piece,* appeared in at least twenty-seven American editions between 1766 and 1831.[6]

The *Aristotle* volumes were essentially descriptive. They abounded in information about the anatomy and physiology of the sexual organs—those of females in particular. (One of the books was a practical handbook about midwifery.) But throughout the series, "Aristotle" made it plain that he considered sex to be both good fun and excellent general therapy. "It eases and lightens the body, clears the mind, comforts the head and senses, and expels melancholy." Sexual abstinence, suggested "Aristotle," could actually do serious harm to a person's health. In the case of men, "sometimes through the omission of this act dimness of sight doth ensue, and giddiness." As for women, continued abstinence could lead to anything from barrenness to an ailment known as "Green Sickness"—characterized by a pale green appearance, breathing difficulties, heart palpitations, and "unusual beatings and small throbbings of the arteries in the temple, neck and back." The Green Sickness could easily be cured, however, by "such copulation as may prove satisfactory to her that is afflicted."[7]

"Aristotle" contended that sexual health demanded not only quantitative but qualitative satisfaction as well. To be worthwhile, sexual intercourse had to be exciting, passionate, even violent. Like the wild beasts, men and women ought to be "furious when they couple. . . . The act of coition should be performed with the greatest ardor and intenseness of desire possible, or else they may as well let it alone."[8]

This ardor was as natural for women as for men. Indeed, "Aristotle" lavished far more attention on female sexuality than he did on male. *The Works of Aristotle,* in the vein of eighteenth-century pornography like John Cleland's *Memoirs of a Woman of Pleasure,* are essentially an eighteenth-century male fantasy about what women are really like. The author suggested, for example, that the onset of female puberty was marked by a fully conscious desire for sexual intercourse:

The inclination of virgins to marriage is to be known by many symptoms: for, when they arrive at ripe age, which is about fourteen or fifteen, their natural purgations begin to flow; and then the blood which can no longer serve for the increase of their bodies does, by its abounding, stir up their minds to venerate [i.e., venery] . . . . Their desire of venereal embraces become very great, and, at some critical junctures almost insupportable. . . . And this strong inclination of theirs may be known by their eager gazing at men, and affecting their company, which sufficiently demonstrates that nature excites them to desire coition.[9]

American interest in the *Works of Aristotle* peaked around the turn of the nineteenth century and then began gradually to fall off. The last known edition of any of the titles appeared in 1831. Its final printing that year can be seen as an event of symbolic significance, a kind of changing-of-the-guard, because in the same year—1831—a New York publisher brought out a short booklet written by J. N. Bolles and entitled *Solitary Vice Considered.* This booklet proved to be the first of a spate of antimasturbation titles that would appear for the rest of the decade—and for a century beyond. The next year saw the first American publication of a seventy-year-old Swiss work (and a classic of sorts on the continent), Samuel A. A. Tissot's *Discourse on Onanism.*[10] In 1833 William A. Alcott, an American, included a long chapter on sexual hygiene in his popular *Young Man's Guide,* and in 1834 Sylvester Graham published the *Lecture to Young Men on Chastity* that he had been delivering in public for two years, and which was to go through ten editions in the next fifteen years. By 1835 articles on masturbation and sexual excess were appearing in such respectable periodicals as the *Boston Medical and Surgical Journal* and the *American Annals of Education.*[11]

The difference between the sexual hygiene literature of the 1830s and the *Works of Aristotle* is obvious at any level. Where "Aristotle" waxed lyric about sex, the writers of the 1830s were tense and suspicious. Where "Aristotle" warned that ill health would result from sexual abstinence, these writers warned that ill health would result from sexual overindulgence. Where he assumed that intense sexual desire was altogether natural, they argued that it was inherently pathological. Where his advice for young people in the throes of lust was to get married as soon as possible, theirs was to eliminate the cause of lust by means of careful attention to diet and regimen. The sexual reformers of the 1830s claimed to base their arguments on scientific observation and not simply on ethical or theological directives. Significantly, most of them were physicians rather than clergymen. (Even Sylvester Graham, the most obvious exception to this rule, encouraged people to refer to him as "Dr. Graham.")[12]

The nature of this shift can be clarified by turning to the one significant work on sexual hygiene that did appear in America during the eighteenth century: *Onania*, the antimasturbation tract published in Boston in 1724. At first glance, *Onania* appears quite similar to the hygienic literature of the 1830s. It was more proscriptive than descriptive; it dealt with the less pleasant aspects of sexuality; and it shared the nineteenth-century writers' obsessive concern with the practice of masturbation.

But a closer reading reveals that the eighteenth-century *Onania* spoke more with the cultural voice of the *Aristotle* titles than with the voice of the "new chastity." For despite all the conviction with which it condemned masturbation, it did not criticize the sexual impulse that led young people to engage in that practice, nor did it deny that there were alternate channels into which the impulse might legitimately be directed. Only masturbation itself was pernicious, and it was pernicious simply because it was a violation of divine decree, natural law, and the stability of the social order. It "hinders marriage, and puts a stop to procreation." It was worse than fornication and adultery because it was not merely a sin "against nature" but a sin "that perverts and extinguishes nature," so that "he who is guilty of it, is laboring at the Destruction of his Kind, and in a manner strikes at the Creation itself." For this reason God has condemned it as an offense punishable by death. But even if God had remained silent, natural human reason would reach the same conclusion: "When we reflect on the End of Marriage [that is, procreation] in all countries, and in all Societies . . . natural Religion, and our own Reason would instruct us, that to destroy that End, must be very offensive to God, if there is one."[13] According to *Onania*, the purely physiological consequences of masturbation were serious, but they were merely the incidental indications that self-abuse was forbidden. Nature's God had devised them in order to demonstrate that there was physiological as well as moral sanctuary to be found in marriage.

The sexual reformers of the 1830s never spoke of divine injunction, and they rarely spoke of natural law. Instead they concentrated almost exclusively on the physiological consequences of masturbation and other violations of sexual hygiene. Sylvester Graham, for instance, proposed simply to set forth "the true physiological and pathological principles which relate to the sexual organization, functions, propensities and passions of man," and to do so "with an accuracy of scientific truth which defies refutation." He did not in any way intend to dispute the biblical doctrine of "sexual continence and purity," but he did propose to demonstrate, "without going out of my way for the purpose," that even the Bible was "founded on the physiological principles established in the constitutional nature of man."[14]

In fact, Graham went well beyond any biblical injunctions on sexual behavior. He argued, for instance, that sex within marriage could be just as harmful to the human constitution as masturbation—especially for young men. It was Graham's contention that only when a man had approached the age of thirty did his body become sufficiently mature to engage in any form of sexual activity. Even when a male did reach his full physiological maturity, he had to restrict sexual expression to a minimum—a single coupling each month for "the healthy and the robust," and less or none at all for the sickly and the sedentary. Marriage provided no sexual sanctuary at all, in other words, because "sexual excess within the pale of wedlock" invariably proved as harmful to the body as masturbation. As Graham bluntly put it,"the mere fact that a man is married to one woman, and is perfectly faithful to her, will by no means prevent the evils which flow from venereal excess."[15]

The anonymous author of *Onania,* on the other hand, went out of his way to stress the sexual freedom available to a married couple. He spoke of the married state as "a Provision for Incontinence in either sex," and a "lawful refuge to all who . . . find themselves incapable of remaining without Sin." While conceding that "there is a decorum to be observ'd as to the Marriage-Bed," he denied that any breach of this decorum could be as serious as a single act of self-pollution. Whatever a married man might do in bed with his wife, or to her, "no branch of it could have any affinity with the Sin of Onan." Where Graham argued that marital excess was as bad as masturbation or even adultery, the author of *Onania* insisted that the best insurance against committing either of these offenses was "carnal copulation, and even the frequent practice of it."[16]

In places *Onania* reads as if it had been written chiefly as an advertisement for marriage. The author often seems to condemn masturbation less out of any real sense that it was dangerous than out of a suspicion that the practice might be providing young men with sufficient sexual relief that marriage was losing its appeal for them. (Historians have pointed out that eighteenth-century England was faced with an increasing surplus of women; indeed, it was at this time that the word "spinster" was coming to assume its modern meaning. It is possible that under these circumstances there would be good reason to advertise the felicities of married life and to attack any alternatives that threatened to subvert it—including the "alternative" of masturbation.) In any case, like the *Aristotle* volumes, *Onania* recommended that people marry young: "Early marriage would be a means of preventing many of those mischiefs, and the Disgrace which oftentimes the Guilty this way bring upon themselves and Families."

The "disgrace" to which this writer alluded was the possibility that youthful masturbation would lead to impotence in adulthood. In fact, almost all the physiological woes that masturbation may cause were related to future sexual depletion: habitual self-abuse "so forces and weakens the tender Vessels, that when they come to Manhood, it renders them ridiculous to women." Indeed, many masturbators were not "able to touch a woman, but *ad primum labiorium contactum semen emittent* [they ejaculate at the first contact with the vaginal lips]." In characteristically eighteenth-century fashion, *Onania* reduced an ostensibly ethical problem to a matter of social embarrassment and "disgrace." Such impotent men, it concluded, were "a jest to others, and a Torment to themselves."[17]

In stressing sexual impotence and loss of desire as the unfortunate consequences of masturbation, the author of *Onania* obviously assumed that desire and potency were healthy conditions. He agreed that sexual *activity* had to be restricted to the marriage bed, but he accepted the idea that lust itself was a perfectly natural impulse to feel—and to satisfy. "All of both Sexes," he wrote in a passage strongly reminiscent of *Aristotle's Master Piece,* "from a natural Instinct, when arrived to the Years of Puberty, and enjoy their full Health and Strength, have amorous Motions." If these "motions" were not acted out, then "for want of a natural Stream, they are over-run into unnatural Practices." If young persons were not permitted to marry shortly after puberty, then "as the Stream is dammed up . . . it doth and will rage the more, and a vent one way or other it will and must have."[18]

Sylvester Graham could not have disagreed more completely. In his eyes intense or persistent sexual desire was neither healthy nor natural. Graham frequently spoke of desire in terms of "aching sensibility," as if it were something painful and unnatural, like a fever or a toothache. He noted that the nerves associated with the sexual organs were, "in their natural state, entirely destitute of animal sensibility," and that good health actually "required such a state of these nerves." Graham never went so far as to claim in so many words that sexual desire, in itself, was actually a diseased state, but he did insist that people who were really healthy could easily "subdue their sexual propensities" to the point where they would be wholly free of sexual feeling "for several months in succession." As he added pointedly, "health does not absolutely require that there should ever be an emission of semen from puberty to death."[19]

The operative word here was *health*. Because Graham believed that sexual morality was rooted in the principles of physiology, it followed that sexual self-control could be achieved neither by a stroke of divine grace nor by the direct application of human will, but only by paying close attention to proper hygienic principles. For Graham, a healthy freedom from sexual desire followed directly from the careful regulation of personal regimen, especially dietary practices—just as improper regimen inevitably led to un-naturally intense prurience. In other words, "this [sexual] propensity is more or less powerful and imperious, according as their dietetic and other habits are more or less correct."

In this way Graham refuted the traditional argument that lust was "im-planted in [people] by Nature, and therefore it is right and proper that they should indulge it, to all extent, consistent with matrimonial rights." If people would only adopt "a proper system of diet and general regimen," he argued, they would "so subdue their sexual propensity, as to be able to abstain from connubial commerce, and preserve entire chastity of body, for several months in succession, without the least inconvenience, and with-out separation from their companions." It was specious, Graham continued, to justify frequent sexual activity by claiming that it was the expression of natural human instinct. The urge that was satisfied by such activity, he argued, was not natural at all: it was only "depraved instinct." Men and women who had perverted their natural drives beyond recognition had lost the right of appealing to Nature. "It is a perfect mockery, to talk about our inherent and ungovernable passions, while we take every measure to deprave our instinctive propensities, and to excite our passions, and render them ungovernable and irresistible."[20]

In order to help people resist the temptation of sexual misbehavior, the *Onania,* with its potpourri of biblicism, enlightenment metaphysics, and traditional folklore, recommended a diverse set of preventive and therapeutic measures to be employed separately or in combination. These suggestions began with sincere Christian "repentance" and "mortification" for those who already practiced the vice, and with moral education for those who were still too young to have discovered it. For habitual mas- turbators, *Onania* went on to prescribe a series of "natural Remedies." These included getting out of bed directly upon waking up—"the Bed is too great a Friend to this Sin"; not handling the genitals or thinking about sexual matters ("till you may think of it with more safety, that is when you are married"); meditating on "sad and doleful objects"; employ- ing a "spare diet," though not an abstemious one (especially at the time of the full moon and the new, "for then the whole body is fuller of Mois- ture than at other seasons"); avoiding salty meats ("which you know by the Nature of the word makes men Salacious"); and avoiding "all windy Foods, such as Beans and Pease, [which] puff up the Humour, and make those Parts more turgid."[21] But the most important recommendation of *Onania,* of course, was getting married. Fully one-third of the book was devoted to this single subject: marriage was the best remedy and the "chief Preventive" for masturbation and for every other sexual vice as well.

Sylvester Graham rejected or ignored virtually all these measures. Mar- riage did not cure sexual abuses; it merely transferred them from one arena to another. Even repentance and moral education, however sincere, were nearly worthless, at least in the absence of proper diet and regimen. Graham cited a case in point—the story of a family he had known years earlier, a family "of considerable distinction for their wealth, refinement and piety." Particularly memorable was the lady of the house, "a very paragon of christian propriety. . . especially as a mother." This woman was "unremit- ting in her maternal efforts to imbue the minds of her children with senti- ments of virtue and piety." She taught the children how to pray as soon as they learned how to talk, and as they grew older they were "successively

introduced into religious Infant and Sunday schools and Bible classes."
To "protect" them from "the contaminating influence of other children,"
she even came to employ "private teachers, who cooperated with her
in all her pious plans and measures." Everyone was confident that "such
a system of education" would achieve "the happiest results."

But when Graham happened to renew his acquaintance with this family
after a break of sixteen years, it was only to discover that the children had
grown up ill-tempered and filled with disrespect toward their family and
its ideals. Most upsetting of all, he found that each of them, and especially
the older daughter, was "spiced" with "excessive lasciviousness." When
she found herself alone with a man, the girl "would not only freely allow
him to take improper liberties with her, without the least restraint, but
would even court his dalliance by her lascivious conduct." Upon being
consulted by the girl's parents, who were worried about the state of her
health, Graham "found that she was addicted to the practice of self-
pollution, and had greatly injured herself by it." Moreover, when Graham
confronted her with the fact of her conduct, the girl "declared that she
had no remorse, no compunction on the subject."

"Here, then," Graham mused, "would seem to be a case in which the
very best efforts of a pious mother had entirely failed of their object."
But there was a single "radical defect" in all those efforts, a defect that
had "completely nullified every good measure." For all the woman's
good intentions, she had "wholly disregarded the relations between the
bodies and the souls of her children—between their dietetic habits and
their moral character." At every meal she had served them "highly seasoned
flesh-meat, rich pastry, and every other kind of rich and savory food, and
condiments in abundance, together with strong coffee and tea, and perhaps occasionally a glass of wine." It was, therefore, no wonder that her
children had become remorseless masturbators: "the result was just what
was reasonably to be expected." Pious and affectionate though she was,
she had become an "active agent in the destruction of her children."[22]

Having demonstrated by this sorry tale that moral education was use-
less in the absence of proper dietary practices, Graham reported another,
happier story to demonstrate that simply dietary reform was capable
of soothing the sexual drive. This story concerned a "highly respectable"
lawyer and his two young sons. As the lawyer himself described the situation in a letter to Graham, he had been in the habit of serving animal food

to the boys from the time of their infancy. When they had reached the age of two and four respectively, their health had become "quite delicate"; even more alarming, both children showed signs of being sexually excitable. It had been the lawyer's custom to awaken the boys each night and "let them urinate, to prevent their wetting the bed." But whenever he did so, it was invariably to find them "affected with priapism [erection]." This also happened whenever the two-year-old sat in his mother's lap; on these occasions "the little fellow manifested an ardor in hugging and kissing her, which had all the appearance of real wantonness." The scene "was often carried so far as actually to embarrass her, when others were present." The same thing generally took place when the little boy caressed other females, the lawyer added, "but when he was in my lap, and hugging or caressing me, or any other gentleman, there were no such indications."

After this problem had been disturbing him for some time, the lawyer happened to attend a series of lectures delivered by Sylvester Graham, and he decided, as a last resort, to follow Graham's advice and to place his boys on "a simple vegetable diet." The strategy immediately resulted in a total and permanent cure. When the children were awakened to urinate each night, they no longer displayed erections; and while, as the lawyer put it, "our younger son is still fond of being in his mother's lap and caressing her," happily "his priapism on such occasions has entirely disappeared." The lawyer was "perfectly convinced" that the "former wantonness" of the children had been "caused by their free use of flesh-meat" and that this wantonness had been cured by the timely substitution of a vegetable diet.[23]

Meat, spices, sweets, coffee, tea and alcohol: these were the substances that intensified the sexual drive. No one was immune to their effects, whether male or female, married or single, old or young. Such was the practical basis of Graham's injunctions. The belief that diet is able to affect the intensity of the sexual feelings was not, to be sure, original with Sylvester Graham. It was present in the *Onania,* and it had been an accepted element in medical theory and practice for at least 2,000 years. Indeed, the idea that certain foods and other substances possess aphrodiasic qualities—that they are sexual "stimulants"—seems to have attained a widespread currency in many eras and cultures. Graham's vegetarian prescriptions are novel, therefore, only in the way he construed them:

in the exclusive emphasis he placed on them and in the way he incorporated them into a complex and highly resonant theory of human physiology.

NOTES

1. Sylvester Graham, *Lecture to Young Men, on Chastity, intended also for the serious consideration of parents and guardians*, 3rd ed. (Boston, 1837), p. 10. Graham delivered this lecture many times in New York City, Boston, and almost every other city he visited for more than a week: Edith Cole, "Sylvester Graham, Lecturer on the Science of Human Life: The Rhetoric of a Dietary Reformer" (Ph.D. diss., Indiana University, 1975), p. 99.

2. Graham, *Chastity*, pp. 12, 21.

3. Edmund S. Morgan, "The Puritans and Sex," *New England Quarterly*, 15 (1942): 591-607; John Demos, "Families in Colonial Bristol, Rhode Island: An Exercise in Historical Demography," *William and Mary Quarterly*, Third Series, 25 (1968): 56-57; Robert A. Gross, *The Minutemen and Their World* (New York, 1976), pp. 100-101, 181-185; Daniel Scott Smith and Michael S. Hindus, "Premarital Pregnancy in America, 1640-1971: An Overview and Interpretation," *Journal of Interdisciplinary History* 5 (1975): 537-570.

4. Benjamin Franklin, *Autobiography*, ed. Leonard W. Labaree et al. (New Haven, 1964), p. 150.

5. Benjamin Wadsworth, *Unchast Practices Procure Divine Judgments* (Boston, 1716); Mason Locke Weems, *God's Revenge against Adultery* (Baltimore, 1815); Cotton Mather, *The Pure Nazarite* (Boston, 1723); [Anon] *Onania, or the Heinous Sin of Self-Pollution, and All Its Frightful Consequences in Both Sexes, Considered* (Boston, 1724).

6. The four "Aristotle" books were (1) *Aristotle's Master Piece; displaying the Secrets of Nature in the Generation of Man*; (2) *Aristotle's Last Legacy; unfolding the Secrets of Nature respecting the Generation of Man*; (3) *Aristotle's Compleat and Experienced Midwife*; and (4) *Aristotle's Book of Problems*. Aristotle, of course, was hardly the author of these works. While a few passages did date back to classical antiquity—especially in the *Book of Problems*—the prose was generally of seventeenth-century British origin. Any given volume changed considerably from edition to edition. See Otho T. Beall, Jr., *"Aristotle's Master Piece* in America: A Landmark in the Folklore of Medicine," *William and Mary Quarterly*, Third Series, 20 (1963): 207-222. The Aristotle books were first published in England at the end of the seventeenth century. Vern Bullough has similarly noted the contrast between the matter-of-factness of "Aristotle" and the moralism of later nineteenth-century sex hygienists such as J. H. Kellogg. Vern Bullough, "An Early American Sex Manual, or Aristotle Who?" *Early American Literature*, 7 (1973): 236-246.

7. *Aristotle's Book of Problems* (Philadelphia, 1792 ed.), p. 37. The description of the Green Sickness is quoted by Beall from an edition of the *Master*

Piece published in New York in 1788. (Beall, *"Aristotle's Master Piece* in America," p. 216.)

8. *Aristotle's Master Piece* (Philadelphia, 1788), p. 18; *Aristotle's Book of Problems*, p. 37; *Aristotle's Last Legacy* (Philadelphia, 1788), p. 17.

9. *Aristotle's Master Piece*, p. 14. At another point, "Aristotle" makes the same point in verse: "Thus nature to her children is so kind,/that early they those inclinations find,/which prompts them on to propagate mankind. /Hence 'tis a virgin her desires can't smother,/but restless is till she be made a mother." (Quoted Beall, *Aristotle's Master Piece*, p. 218). Aristotle saw women essentially as the physiological twin of men and their anatomical mirror-images (the concavities of the one corresponding to the convexities of the other). As he phrased it in an attempted couplet: "Man and wife are but one right/canonical hermaphrodite" (*Last Legacy*, p. 7). Like other writers of his time, "Aristotle" believed that women as well as men had "seminal vessels" which at the moment of orgasm expelled a "seed." The "seed" of the woman then joined with that of the man and a child was conceived (see the *Last Legacy*, pp. 8-11; the *Master Piece*, pp. 10-11; and the *Experienced Midwife*, pp. 16-17). It was probably this lingering idea of conception that was responsible for the belief, almost universally expressed in nineteenth-century pornography, that women had ejaculations during orgasm. The anonymous author of *My Secret Life* (ca. 1890), for instance, actually retained the belief that female orgasm was required for conception to take place. It is probably no coincidence that he acknowledges having gained his initial information about sex from the "Aristotle" books.

10. Samuel A. Tissot's *L'Onanisme* had been published in French, in Lausanne in 1760, several years after its original appearance in Latin. This work probably achieved such wide circulation in Europe during the late eighteenth century because it was the first "scientific" work on masturbation to be published in a non-Latin version. Earlier works on the subject clearly had been intended for the use of physicians and clergymen; *L'Onanisme* was written for the literate public. A further discussion of this book will be found in Chapter 7.

11. See, for example, the *Boston Medical and Surgical Journal* 12 (1835): 109, 138, and the *American Annals of Education*, series 3, 5 (1835): 211-214. The author of the articles in the former probably was Samuel B. Woodward, who later published a book on the subject, *Hints to the Young, on a subject relating to the Health of Body and Mind* (Boston, 1838). For titles that followed in the 1840s and beyond, see the Bibliography. H. Tristram Englehardt, Jr. has discussed the overall character of the large nineteenth-century literature on masturbation in his article, "The Disease of Masturbation: Values and the Concept of Disease," *Bulletin of the History of Medicine* 48 (1974): 234-248. Englehardt's view that nineteenth-century concepts of masturbation as a disease entity were based on "a general suspicion that sexual activity was debilitating" (p. 239) coincides with my analysis of Graham as a representative figure of his times. A more general description of nineteenth-century beliefs about the causes and treatment of masturbatory "diseases" can be found in John S. Haller and Robin M. Haller, *The Physician and Sexuality in Victorian America* (Urbana, Ill., 1974), pp. 195-211.

12. In a recent article Arthur N. Gilbert has advanced some intriguing hypotheses to explain increasing medical attention to the problem of masturbation. Most evolve from the plausible idea that the nineteenth-century medical profession was attempting to claim—and often being asked to assume—a social and moral prestige well in excess of its technological capabilities. It was thus attracted and almost compelled to make use of artifactual disease categories with useful moral overtones—like masturbation—to bridge uncomfortable gaps in diagnosis and therapeutics. See Arthur N. Gilbert, "Doctor, Patient, and Onanist Diseases in the 19th Century," *Journal of the History of Medicine* 30 (1975): 217-234.

13. *Onania,* p. 8. A somewhat fuller discussion of *Onania* can be found in Stephen Nissenbaum, "Careful Love: Sylvester Graham and the Emergence of Victorian Sexual Theory in America, 1830-1840" (Ph.D. diss., University of Wisconsin, 1968), pp. 11-24.

14. Graham, *Chastity,* pp. 23-24.

15. Ibid., pp. 21, 73.

16. *Onania,* pp. 17, 57-59. Responding at one point to the argument that married couples should abstain from sexual contact at certain times, *Onania* asks "what shall we say to a young couple, both in health, that Live in Peace and Harmony, and have been a considerable time striving to render themselves delightful and endearing to each other? How shall they practice this forbearance, when every Night, naked, they lie in the same bed together . . .?" (p.59).

17. Ibid., pp. 45-46. See also pp. 15-18.

18. *Onania,* pp. 46-47.

19. Graham, *Chastity,* pp. 44, 50, 80; *Lectures on the Science of Human Life,* 2 vols. (Boston, 1839), 2:646.

20. Graham, *Chastity,* pp. 79-81, 86.

21. *Onania,* pp. 33, 41, 44.

22. Graham, *Chastity,* pp. 165-169.

23. Ibid., pp. 176-179.

3. VEGETARIANISM

When Sylvester Graham first propounded his dietary principles in the *Lecture on Chastity,* he became only the second public advocate of vegetarianism in America. The first was an English clergyman named William Metcalfe, who had emigrated with a group of his followers in 1817 to Philadelphia where he established the "Bible Christian Church" on vegetarian principles. The traditional story is that Graham became acquainted with Metcalfe in Philadelphia in 1830, and that it was from this encounter that Graham acquired his own vegetarian leanings. It is possible that the two men did meet—Graham was lecturing in Philadelphia at the time—but it would be silly to attribute Graham's vegetarianism to the influence of an encounter with the English minister. The dietary principles of the two men actually had little in common during this period. Graham's position was based form the beginning on purely physiological considerations, while Metcalfe initially derived his vegetarianism from an interpretation of certain Biblical texts.[1]

In fact, Graham did not base his views on any of the numerous vegetarian sources available to him. The long history of vegetarianism includes several distinct traditions, and Metcalfe's biblical position represents just one of these. Vegetarian theory actually antedates Christianity, originating in classical antiquity. The Greek mystic Pythagorus (sixth century B.C.) and the Neoplatonist Porphyry (third century A.D.) both wrote extensive treatises on the subject. The vegetarianism of both these men stemmed from a belief that human life was poised precariously between two poles, the divine and the bestial, and that people's spiritual destiny depended on which of these two poles they most closely approached in their daily lives. By this philosophy, it was brutalizing to kill and eat living creatures, and those who did so were thereby placing their spirituality in jeopardy. The eating of vegetable foods, on the other hand, reinforced the higher and more rational element in human nature. In neither case was the purely physiological effect of diet a matter of any consequence. As a follower of Graham noted in 1838 in an attempt to distinguish Pythogorean vegetarianism from the Grahamite variety, the former was not primarily intended to make men "better, or more healthy, or longer-lived *animals,*" but to make them "better rationals, more truly noble and godlike."[2]

A similar position, although its format was Christian rather than pagan, was taken late in the seventeenth century by Thomas Tryon (1634-1703), an Englishman whose book *The Way to Health* temporarily converted to vegetarianism the young Benjamin Franklin who encountered Tryon's book while living in London in 1722.[3] In Tryon's view, both man's "strong inclination after Flesh" and "his making so light and small a matter" of killing animals to satisfy this inclination demonstrate "what Principle has got the Dominion in him." Had humanity "continued in the pure law of God," it "would have been far from oppressing , killing, or eating the Flesh and Blood of the Beasts, which was not allowed him in the beginning."[4] The resemblance between these views and those of Pythagorus is no accident: Tryon was also the author of a book on the Pythagorean philosophy.[5]

On the other hand, there is a purely humanitarian element in Tryon's vegetarianism—an open sympathy for the suffering of the murdered beasts—that is independent of both his Pythagoreanism and of the biblicism in which it is couched. (One chapter in Tryon's book is entitled "The Voice of the Dumb: or the complaints of the Creatures, expostulating with Man, touching the cruel Usages they suffer from him.")[6] This humanitarian spirit emerged a century later in the writings of a group of English writers, the first "modern" vegetarians, including John Oswald (*The Cry of Nature,* 1791), George Nicholson (*On the Conduct of Man to Inferior Animals,* 1797), Joseph Ritson (*Abstinence from flesh, a Moral Duty,* 1802), and Sir Richard Phillips (an 1811 article in the *Medical Journal*). By emphasizing the animal suffering that inevitably accompanied a diet of flesh, these works tended to ignore not only the physiological but even the moral effects of meat-eating on persons who practiced it. In this sense they bore even less resemblance than did Pythagoreanism to Graham's brand of vegetarianism.[7] In all of Graham's writing on the subject there is not one word that could be described as humanitarian in this sense.

There are, to be sure, books in which the physical effects of meat on the human system are discussed, books whose primary concern *is* to make men healthier "animals." But, these books are not, strictly speaking, vegetarian in their position. They belong to an altogether different genre: the manual of hygiene. Like vegetarian treatises, hygiene manuals date back to classical antiquity—there is one, for instance, by the Roman physician Galen (130-200 A.D.)—but it was only much later that such works achieved any significant popular appeal. About the time of the Renaissance, people began to feel that the duration of human life was, like so much else in the world, subject to direct human control. In response to this feeling there emerged a body of literature which contended that the most effective means of achieving longer life was to pay careful attention to diet and regimen.

Easily the most popular of these hygienic works was Luigi Cornaro's *Discourses on a Sober and Temperate Life*. First published in 1558, *Discourses* was soon translated into several languages and reprinted sporadically well into the nineteenth century. (Sylvester Graham himself brought out an American edition of the book in 1832.) Cornaro was a Venetian nobleman, born in 1467, whose gluttonous habits had brought him near the point of death by the time he was forty. He was rescued from the abyss, however, by what he termed a "reformation"—not exactly an unfamiliar term during the early sixteenth century—in his diet and regimen. This reformation completely restored his health, and thanks to it Cornaro lived to the age of ninety-eight. *Discourses*, composed in several sections when he was a very old man, was intended to serve both as an exposition of the dietary principles he had come to practice and as a kind of living testimony to the fact that he had retained complete possession of his mental faculties until the end.

Cornaro based his dietary rules on the classical principle that the world consists of four basic elements apportioned to provide perfect balance, and also on Galen's adaptation of this principle to human life—the idea that the human body "is no more than a harmonious combination of the same four elements."[8] It was therefore necessary, Cornaro reasoned, that the body "be preserved and maintained by the very same order" as the world outside it. Since food alone failed to provide all four elements—air, for instance—it followed that habitual gluttony would provoke an imbalance in nature's harmonious arrangement. Regularity and moderation, then, were the key to a long and healthy life. "Whoever leads a sober and regular life, and commits no excess in diet, can suffer but very little from disorders of any other kind, or external accidents."[9]

In the light of these principles, it is not surprising that despite his concern for the effects of diet upon health, Cornaro was no vegetarian. From his point of view, to renounce meat altogether would be as immoderate as to eat meat alone. The diet that had prevented his own dissolution, and which he recommended to others, included "veal, kid, and mutton . . . poultry of every kind . . . partridge, and other birds, such as thrushes." ("I likewise eat fish," he added.) "All these things are fit for an old man," he boasted in language that proved obviously embarrassing to his nineteenth-century Grahamite editors, "and, therefore, he ought to be content with them."[10] What preserved his own health, Cornaro insisted throughout *Discourses,* was that he consumed only such food and drink as "agreed with my constitution," and that he consumed it only in "the quantity I knew I could digest." Specifically, this meant that he permitted himself twelve ounces of food per day, and fourteen ounces of wine—new wine only, he noted, since aged wine invariably made him ill.[11]

Cornaro's dietary rules were restrictive only in a quantitative way: They enjoined people from eating "a greater quantity of any kind of food, even of that which agrees with them, than what their stomachs can easily digest." But when his rules touched on the *kinds* of food to be eaten, they were quite permissive. An individual might eat whatever agreed with his "constitution." Those persons "with whom nothing disagrees, are not bound to observe any rule but that relating to the quantity and not to the quality, of their food."[12]

In the course of the eighteenth century a number of physicians, most of them men of considerable eminence, followed Cornaro's lead and composed manuals of personal hygiene which were nontechnical and designed specifically for the literate public. Among those published in English, either originally or in translation, were George Cheyne's *Essay of Health and Long Life* (1724), Samuel Tissot's *Advice to the People on their Health* (1762), Christopher Hufeland's *Art of Prolonging Life* (1797), Bernard Faust's *Catechism of Health* (1797), and Thomas Beddoes' *Hygeia* (1802). Similar books were sometimes written by men who were not physicians, such as Sir John Sinclair (the well-known Scottish lawyer and agricultural theorist who published *The Code of Health and Longevity* in 1807.) In addition, there were several books intended for public consumption which provided lists of home remedies (including diet and regimen) for every possible disease. The most popular of these were the Reverend John Wesley's *Primitive Physick* (1747)—a book that was reprinted more often, and probably reached a wider public, than any of Wesley's religious titles—and William Buchan's *Domestic Medicine* (1769).

All these works emphasized the necessity for moderation in diet, especially for the sick or infirm, but none recommended abstaining from meat. In fact, it was the generally accepted view at this time that even though meat might be more difficult to digest, it provided greater and more easily accessible nourishment than other types of food. Because it more nearly resembled the composition of the human body that assimilated it, meat needed to undergo a less radical transformation in the digestive process. For this reason, if for no other, it was not possible for the hygienicists (as it was for such writers as Thomas Tryon or for the humanitarian vegetarians) to recommend that people abstain from animal food.

Such a belief in the digestibility of meat, and the superior nourishment it afforded, was so pervasive that it was accepted even by the single eighteenth-century hygienicist who most closely approached a theoretical vegetarianism. George Cheyne, whose *Essay of Health and Long Life* was the first of the popular eighteenth-century hygiene manuals, admitted he occasionally "indulged a conjecture" that animal food was "not intended for human creatures." Cheyne quickly added, however, that this conjecture did not apply to the present condition of mankind but only to "the original frame of our nature, and design of our creation." Cheyne did eventually adopt a vegetarian diet for himself, but since he weighed more than 400 pounds when he did so, it is unlikely that he took the step simply in response to his philosophical conjectures. In fact, Cheyne recommended animal food to those in good health, and like the other hygienic writers of the century, he devoted a large section of his *Essay* to a discussion of the best cuts of meat and the best ways of cooking them.[13]

The belief that animal food was superior to vegetable in the quality and the accessibility of its nourishment lingered into the nineteenth century, a period during which the interest in hygiene grew widespread and intense. It was probably this belief that delayed the emergence of an unambiguous "physiological" vegetarianism, at least in America, until the 1830s—despite the fact that a number of hygienic writers, impelled by their involvement in the burgeoning temperance movement, were coming to develop a suspicion of animal food almost as intense as their aversion to liquor. These writers invariably ended their diatribes against meat with the reluctant admission that man was, after all, an "omniverous" creature. Like Luigi Cornaro, they prescribed dietary rules that were more quantitative than qualitative, even when they took the Italian to task, along with the eighteenth-century hygienists, for being far too tolerant of items such as wine and liquor.[14]

Nowhere is this ambivalence toward animal food more apparent than in Edward Hitchcock's *Dyspepsy Forestalled* (1830). Hitchcock, a well-known clergyman and geologist—professor of chemistry at Amherst College in 1830, and later president of the college—was an early temperance advocate. His books originated as a series of lectures he delivered to the Amherst student body. Hitchcock was himself a long-time "dyspeptic"—the term at this time was a catch-all for a whole series of chronic "nervous" complaints that in one way or another managed to affect the digestive apparatus—and he composed the lectures in order to stem what he called "the premature prostration and early decay of students and professional men in our country."

While Hitchcock unequivocally condemned the use of alcohol in any form (along with coffee, tea, and tobacco), none of the nine elaborate dietary rules he enumerated actually proscribed the eating of meat. The furthest he went in that direction was to suggest that "sedentary persons [e.g., students and professional men] should not use animal food more than once a day." For such people, Hitchcock argued, "the effect of such animal food, is to produce too much excitement in the system, and to urge on the powers of life too fast."[15]

On the other hand, Hitchcock made it clear that he was deeply suspicious of the effects of meat even on those who were not "sedentary." He claimed, for example, that animal food was "much more unfavourable to the free operations of the mind, than vegetable," and he quoted one writer who argued that vegetable food "tends to preserve a delicacy of feeling, a liveliness of imagination, and acuteness of judgment, seldom enjoyed by those who live principally on meat." He even went so far as to suggest, quite tentatively, that older people and children, whose constitutions were naturally weak, "would probably do best, in general, to confine themselves to vegetables alone."[16]

But even though Hitchcock clearly suspected that animal food was harmful to the human system, he nevertheless felt compelled to admit that it was a necessary part of any healthy diet. Marshalling with obvious reluctance all the ideas that remained current in the 1820s, he argued that it was apparent from the anatomical structure of man's teeth that he "was intended to feed upon [both] vegetables and animals"; from the chemical composition of meat "that some animal food is necessary to the support of life"; and from the physiological process of human digestion "that animal food is more nutritive and stimulating, [and] will sustain life longer" than vegetable food. Because Hitchcock continued to accept the idea that meat had a definite therapeutic value, he was even forced to "admit"—the word was his own—that "persons in feeble health may, under certain circumstances, require the constant and almost exclusive use of animal food."[17]

As for the rest of Hitchcock's dietetic rules, they are all concerned either with the conditions under which meals should be eaten ("slowly . . . with the mind free and the feelings cheerful," and never "while much fatigued") or with the allowable quantity of food ("very moderate" at any one meal, and "only three" meals per day—although this last was designed exclusively for "literary men"). Gluttony, Hitchcock insisted, was as harmful as drunkenness; and the effects on the intellectual and moral faculties produced by "excess in eating" were similar to those produced by "excess in drinking." "How much is there to choose," he asked, "between the swinish insensibility of the glutton, and the frantic ravings of the drunkard?" Gluttony, however, was a quantitative sin, and not a qualitative one, and by comparing it to drunkenness Hitchcock did not intend to suggest that one became a glutton by eating any particular kind of food. In fact, at one point Hitchcock insisted, in a statement at which even Luigi Cornaro, for all his permissiveness, probably would have winced, that "there is scarcely any article of food that may not be digested with comfort, even by a weak stomach, provided the quantity be not too large."

For all his vegetarian leanings, Hitchcock was too prudent to fly in the face of the accepted scientific opinion of his time and to claim that animal food was unnecessary to sustain human life. But within a very few years, after the name of Sylvester Graham had become famous, he could have made just such a claim.[18]

The first serious scientific effort to demonstrate that a vegetable diet was not necessarily debilitating was made early in the nineteenth century by an English physician named William Lambe. Lambe had long been suffering from a variety of chronic diseases when he decided, in 1806, to investigate what would happen to his health if he temporarily abandoned the use of animal food. The results of the experiment were so encouraging he decided to continue it on a permanent basis. Writing of his experience in the third person, Lambe later reported that "he never found the smallest real ill-consequences from this change. He sank neither in flesh, strength, nor in spirits. . . . He has rather gained than lost flesh. He has experienced neither indigestion nor flatulence . . . nor has the stomach suffered from any vegetable matter, though unchanged by any culinary art or uncorrected by condiments."[19]

After trying the same diet on several of his patients, Lambe published the results of his experiment as *Additional Reports on the Effects of a Peculiar Regimen, in Cases of Cancer, Scrofula, Consumption, Asthma, and other Chronic Diseases* in 1815. This book contained just what its title suggests: an empirical demonstration that vegetable diet provided enough energy and nutriment to sustain human life, and that far from being debilitating, it was in fact wholly beneficial in cases of certain chronic complaints. Nowhere in the *Additional Reports* did Lambe recommend a vegetable diet to persons in good health, or claim that animal food had any ill-effects on such people. The book was not, in other words, a tract for vegetarianism. Nevertheless, by purporting to refute the single most convincing physiological argument against vegetarianism, it provided a firm position for those who might care to produce such a tract.[20]

While Lambe's publications do not appear to have attained wide circulation outside of medical circles, his vegetarian experiment was known, at least in England, to a small but highly articulate circle of individuals who were not medical professionals. Lambe's experiment probably appealed to these people, all of them radicals, because of their fondness for the writings of Jean Jacques Rousseau, and especially his great work *Emile*. (Rousseau himself was not a vegetarian, and he did not recommend vegetarianism to others, but he did emphasize the desirability of a "natural" diet—food that was "plain and simple," devoid of such "strong flavors" as salt or alcohol.)[21]

One of this small group of Englishmen, a "habitual invalid" named John Frank Newton, restored his health by adopting Lambe's "peculiar regimen," and in 1811 published a vegetarian tract, *The Return to Nature*. Composed with Rousseauian rhetoric and dedicated to Lambe, Newton's pamphlet achieved no great popularity, but it did have one significant result: it converted Newton's friend, the radical poet and essayist Percy Bysshe Shelley, to vegetarianism. Shelley became a vegetarian in 1813 at the age of twenty-one, and when he published his long poem *Queen Mab* that same year, he

appended a long footnote in which he attacked animal diet. This footnote
was published separately the next year, in a small edition, as *A Vindication
of Natural Diet.* In his pamphlet Shelley utilized a variety of arguments—
moral, anatomical, medical, and economic—but his basic position was an
extension of Rousseau's. (In addition, Shelley quoted extensively from
Newton's *Return to Nature,* and he referred occasionally to the work of
Lambe.)[22]

Shelley proclaimed that animal food was "at the root of all evil." According to his dietary version of the Eden legend, human beings in their
original state of innocence neither ate nor craved meat, but "at some
distant period man forsook the path of nature, and sacrificed the purity
and happiness of his being to unnatural appetites." In Shelley's view this
transformation (represented symbolically by Prometheus's gift of fire—
the instrument of cooking) was a brand of original sin, and from it stemmed
"the depravity of the physical and moral nature of man." "From this moment," Shelley claimed, "his vitals were devoured by the vulture of disease."
Besides leading to physical decay, meat-eating was the cause of "all vice"—
an intriguing list which included tyranny, superstition, commerce, and in-
equality. It was in fact the prevalence of animal diet that spawned all the
most disgraceful episodes in human history, including two that possessed
particular significance for people in Shelley's own generation: the revolutionary Terror in France (if the Parisians had only "satisfied their hunger
at the ever-furnished table of vegetable nature," they would never have
"lent their brutal suffrage to the proscription list of Robespierre); and
the murderous tyranny of Napoleon Bonaparte (had he "descended from
a race of vegetable eaters," the French leader would not have had "either
the inclination or the power to ascend the throne of the Bourbons").
"Pregnant indeed with inexhaustible calamity," Shelley concluded, "is
the renunciation of instinct."[23]

The single hope for the human race lay in what Newton had called a
"return to nature." Only by recapturing its primal and instinctive drives
through a renunciation of animal food and strong drink could the physical
and moral health of humanity be restored. But once such a renunciation
was made, argued Shelley, debility and disease would give way to buoyant
strength, and vice to bucolic innocence. On a physical level, "old age would
be our last and our only malady." On a moral level, vegetable diet would
lead to nothing less than a thorough purification of political and social life.
All "excessive complication of political relations" would be "simplified,"

and pastoral pursuits would replace "commerce, with all its vices, selfishness, and corruption." A vegetable diet would thus achieve "the object of all political speculation"—a state of society "where all the energies of man shall be directed to his solid happiness." It would produce this radical effect because, unlike any "mere reform of legislation," dietary reform "strikes at the root of all evil"—at "the furious passions and evil propensities of the human heart."[24]

Here, finally, in the second decade of the nineteenth century, was a theory of vegetarianism that was forceful, unequivocal, and based on physiological considerations. More nearly than anyone else, it was Shelley who anticipated Graham's position. This was not fortuitous. Like Graham, Shelley was profoundly suspicious of the emergent capitalist order and the threat it posed to traditional social values. Like Graham, too, he associated the new order with physical as well as moral decay. Finally, both Shelley and Graham attributed both types of decay to the introduction of animal food into the human diet.

The great romantic radical poet and the crotchety "prophet of bran bread and pumpkins": it was an improbable conjunction. But if Shelley was regarded as a dangerous revolutionary, the similarity of his ideas to Graham's may serve to emphasize the radical message that was always implicit in Graham's work—along with the reactionary strain that tinged Shelley's radicalism.

This double ambiguity is revealed in the nature of Shelley's notorious attacks on monogamous marriage. In Shelley's view, marriage itself was just another in the long series of unnatural institutions that civilization had forced upon humanity. In the long footnote on vegetarianism he appended to *Queen Mab,* Shelley argued that "the mistakes cherished by society respecting the connexion of the sexes"—that is, marriage—had helped contribute, along with animal diet, "to the mass of human evil." And *Queen Mab* itself was a revolutionary poetic manifesto whose vitriolic assault on marriage and religion influenced later reformers such as Robert Dale Owen and Frances Wright—the very people, ironically, whose "efforts to encourage illicit and promiscuous commerce between the sexes" provoked Sylvester Graham to publish his *Lecture on Chastity.*[25]

But as Graham's own use of the word "commerce" in the last sentence suggests, this irony is more apparent than real. For Shelley's critique of marriage was tinged with the fear of sexuality that Graham was the first to articulate publicly. Shelley blamed marriage not only, as one might expect, for "the misery and diseases of celibacy," but also for the prevalence of "unenjoying prostitution" and, most surprisingly, for the "premature arrival of puberty" in the modern world. As we shall see, several of Graham's own most devoted disciples ended up by adopting Shelley's position on marriage—as open advocates of free love. In the final analysis, Shelley's sexual radicalism was born of the same impulse as Graham's prudery.

Because of Shelley's unconventional views on social questions, his equally unconventional personal life, and the somewhat unsavory reputation that both of these earned him, it is probable that Graham had not read the *Vindication* when he was formulating his own vegetarian position.[26] But even if he had read it, it would have provided only an attitude, and not an explanation. Shelley furnished the idea that man's health and well-being had been destroyed by animal food, but he did not delineate, or even suggest, the actual physiological process by which that destruction took place. Shelley was willing to admit that this process had not yet been discovered; but he did not doubt that it existed and could be described. "Should ever a physician be born with the genius of Locke," Shelley predicted, "I am persuaded that he might trace all bodily and mental derangements to our unnatural habits, as clearly as that philosopher has traced all knowledge to sensation."[27] Although Sylvester Graham was neither a physician nor a genius, that was precisely the connection he attempted to trace.

NOTES

1. Later in his life William Metcalfe's interests seem to have broadened. In 1850 he founded the American Vegetarian Society and edited its magazine, *The American Vegetarian*, which utilized a wide variety of arguments against meat-eating. For information about Metcalfe's career, see Charles W. Forward, *Fifty Years of Food Reform: A History of the Vegetarian Movement in England* (London and Manchester, 1898), pp. 13-15; and Gerald Carson, *Cornflake Crusade* (New York, 1957), pp. 16-19, 265. See also Lafayette B. Mendel, "Some Historical Aspects of Vegetarianism," *Popular Science Monthly* 64 (1904): 462-463; and William A. Alcott, *Vegetable Diet* (Boston, 1838), pp. 214-215.

2. Alcott, *Vegetable Diet*, p. 212. For an analysis of Pythagorean and Porphyrean vegetarianism, see Esme Wynne-Tyson's introduction to *Porphyry on Abstinence from Animal Food* ([London], 1965). Porphyry's teacher, Plotinus, was also a vegetarian, and on similar grounds.

3. The episode is reported in Benjamin Franklin's *Autobiography*, ed. Leonard W. Labaree et al (New Haven, 1964), pp. 63, 87-89. An interesting analysis of this passage can be found in Richard L. Bushman, "On the Uses of Psychology: Conflict and Conciliation in Benjamin Franklin," *History and Theory* 5 (1966): 225-240. It is possible that the title of Franklin's *The Way to Wealth* was intended as an allusion to Tryon.

4. Thomas Tryon, *The Way to Health*, 3rd ed. (London, 1697), p. 232.

5. Thomas Tryon, *Pythagorus his mystick Philosophy reviv'd; or, the mystery of dreams unfolded* (London, 1691). See also A. Cocchi, *The Pythagorean diet of vegetables only* (London, 1745).

6. Tryon, *Way to Health*, pp. 333-347.

7. Forward, *Fifty Years of Food Reform*, pp. 6-9. Even though Phillips's article appeared in a medical publication, it did not employ any physiological arguments.

8. Luigi Cornaro, *Discourses on a Sober and Temperate Life*, ed. John Burdell (New York, 1842), p. 26. Burdell was a Grahamite, as he makes clear in his notes to the book. For a description of his own principles, see ibid., p. 33 n.

9. Cornaro, *Discourses*, pp. 21, 26. See also p. 40.

10. Ibid., p. 75. Burdell expressed his embarrassment in a number of footnotes that attempted to apologize for Cornaro's occasional lapses from the true principles of human physiology.

11. Ibid., pp. 14, 16, 100-101. For a discussion of Cornaro's diet, see William B. Walker, "Luigi Cornaro, A Renaissance Writer on Personal Hygiene," *Bulletin of the History of Medicine*, 28 (1954): 525-534.

12. Cornaro, *Discourses*, p. 35. Burdell appends a footnote to this passage in which he insists that some foods only *seem* to agree with the stomach but in reality do not, so that Cornaro's recommendation "will not always be a safe rule to follow" (p. 156). Other passages to which Burdell takes exception—most of them concerning Cornaro's partiality to wine—can be found on pp. 14, 27, and 102.

13. George Cheyne, An *Essay of Health and Long Life* (London, 1724), p. 84. The reference to Cheyne's weight can be found in Alcott, *Vegetable Diet*, p. 90, and in the *Journal of Health* (Philadelphia), 1 (1829): 231. Alcott insists that Cheyne was a principled vegetarian, but I have found no evidence for this, and there certainly is none in his most popular book.

14. See, for example, W. Nisbet, *A Practical Treatise on Diet* (London, 1801); Thomas Trotter, *View of the Nervous Temperament* (London, 1807); J. M. Adair, *An Essay on Diet and Regimen* (London, 1812); William Kitchiner, *The Art of Invigorating and Prolonging Life*, 2nd ed. (London, 1821; Philadelphia, 1823); [Anon.] *Le catechisme de la medicine physiologique* (Paris, 1824); Charles Londe, *Nouveaux elemens d'hygiene*, 2 vols. (Paris, 1827); John Ayrton Paris, *An Essay on Diet* (London, 1826); C. Pavet de Courtelle, *Hygiene des colleges et des maisons d'education* (Paris, 1827); Charles Whitlaw, *New Medical Discoveries* (London, 1829); and S. W. Avery, *The Dyspeptic's Monitor* (New York, 1829).

15. Edward Hitchcock, *Dyspepsy Forestalled*, 2nd ed., (Northampton, 1831),

VEGETARIANISM / 51

pp. 13, 97. Here too the assumption is not that meat is actually harmful, but that it provides more energy than "sedentary" persons generally require.

16. Ibid., pp. 98-99. Even here Hitchcock uses qualifiers such as "probably" and "in general."

17. Ibid., pp. 94-99.

18. Ibid., pp. 73, 183. See also S. W. Avery, *The Dyspeptic's Monitor.*

19. Quoted in Forward, *Fifty Years of Food Reform,* pp. 7-8.

20. Lambe had published an earlier, more tentative work in 1809: *Reports on the Effects of a peculiar regimen on scirrhous tumours and cancerous ulcers.* By the 1830s, Lambe had in fact become a champion of vegetarianism, and he even carried on a correspondence with Sylvester Graham during these years. Only his earlier work, however, is relevant here, and that work appears to have been wholly unknown in America. Hitchcock, for instance, does not include it in the extensive bibliography appended to *Dyspepsy Forestalled.* In addition to the valuable service already mentioned, Lambe's work also helped give currency to what would soon become a standard argument for vegetarianism—that the human digestive tract and dental apparatus were structurally unsuited to a carnivorous diet. For a discussion of this and other issues in the nineteenth-century debate over the relative merits of vegetable and animal diets, ses James C. Whorton, "Tempest in a Flesh-Pot: The Formulation of a Physiological Rationale for Vegetarianism," *Journal of the History of Medicine,* 32 (1977): 115-139.

21. "Our first food is milk," Rousseau wrote; "we only become accustomed by degrees to strong flavors; at first we dislike them. Fruit, vegetables, herbs, and then fried meat without salt or seasoning, form the feasts of primitive man.... Preserve the child's primitive tastes as long as possible; let his food be plain and simple, let strong flavors be unknown to his palate...." Jean Jacques Rousseau, *Emile* (1762; Dutton Everyman ed., London, 1911), p. 116.

22. Shelley wrote about John Frank Newton's *Return to Nature* (1811) that "it is from that book, and from the conversation of its excellent and enlightened author, that I have derived the materials which I here present to the public." Percy Bysshe Shelley, *A Vindication of Natural Diet,* in Shelley, *Works in Verse and Prose,* 8 vols. (London, 1880), 6:16.

23. Ibid., 6: 5, 7, 13, 14.

24. Ibid., 6:15, 17. "In the history of modern times," Shelley continued, "the avarice of commercial monopoly, no less than the ambition of weak and wicked chiefs, seems to have fomented the universal discord which has come to pervade society. Let it ever be remembered, that it is the direct influence of commerce to make the interval between the richest and the poorest man wider and more unconquerable.... The odious and disgusting aristocracy of wealth, is built upon the ruins of all that is good in chivalry or republicanism" (p. 18).

25. Footnote to Shelley's *Queen Mab,* quoted in Alcott, *Vegetarian Diet,* p. 199. The passage attacking marriage, incidentally, was included only in the original version of the *Vindication,* printed as a footnote to *Queen Mab.* When the tract was published separately the following year, Shelley dropped the entire paragraph—presumably to render the text more palatable.

26. In its pamphlet form, the tract had only a tiny circulation in England. The only place Graham possibly could have encountered it would have been in an edition of *Queen Mab*, and for a variety of reasons—among them Graham's apparent lack of interest in literature—it is unlikely he read the poem. On the other hand, Newton's *Return to Nature* was reviewed (briefly and not wholly favorably) in the *Journal of Health*, which was published at Philadelphia from 1829 to 1833, so there is good reason to believe Graham probably read it. See *Journal of Health*, 3 (1832): 232-233.

27. Shelley, *Works*, 6:13.

4. PHYSIOLOGY

It is clear that even though vegetarianism had a long history, and even though animal diet was increasingly suspect in some circles during the late 1820s. Sylvester Graham in no way found his position ready-made. On the other hand, he did not construct it out of thin air. What Graham did was to join the vegetarian sentiments he shared with men like Percy Bysshe Shelley, Edward Hitchcock, and William Metcalfe, with a conception of physiology he derived from the work of two prominent French medical theorists, François Broussais (1772-1832) and Xavier Bichat (1771-1802). It is no accident that despite his lack of medical training, Graham happened to read and digest these highly technical writings. He did so because of two circumstances which intersected in his career during the years 1829 to 1831: the state of medical development in the city of Philadelphia and the progress of the temperance movement. The first gave Graham the opportunity to encounter the two French medical theorists, and the second provided him with the predisposition to adopt their views as his own.

When Graham first came to Philadelphia shortly before 1830, that city, with its two medical schools, dominated American medicine as it had previously dominated American commerce. Like its economic prosperity, its medical preeminence dated from the middle of the eighteenth century; and if the one was exemplified by Benjamin Franklin, the other was exemplified, a generation later, by a man of similar versatility—Dr. Benjamin Rush. Like Franklin an active participant in the American Revolution and a signer of the Declaration of Independence, it was Rush who was largely responsible for the acceptance, in America, of an unfamiliar system of physiology and pathology. This system itself later came to be replaced and discredited, but it exerted an influence that, in Philadelphia at least, was still perceptible late in the 1820s.

By the middle of the eighteenth century, the so-called humoral physiology, which had been widely accepted from the time of Galen, was thoroughly out of fashion,[1] but it had not been replaced by any widely accepted substitute, and medicine was in a state of extreme flux. The need to explain the nature of disease, and of life itself, led medical theorists in a variety of new directions. One of the more significant of these new ideas stressed the importance of the nervous system. As far back as the middle of the seventeenth century, the Englishman Francis Glisson (1597-1677) had defined the special property of living tissue as "irritability." At the close of that century Friedrich Hoffman (1660-1742), a German, suggested that "moving fibres" are characterized by a certain degree of action or "tone," which can be either increased to generate a "spasm" or diminished to produce a state of "atony."

It was this idea that the Scottish physician William Cullen (1712-1790) adopted as the basis for a general theory of health and disease. Cullen believed that the nervous system was the basis of life, and that it was the source of those regulatory powers that traditionally had been ascribed to the four humors. For this reason any significant increase or diminution of nervous energy, whether provoked by external or internal causes, induced conditions of spasm or debility in the muscles and blood vessels. According to Cullen, therefore, the aim of any treatment should be either to increase the flow of nervous energy by means of drugs and stimulating diet, or to reduce the flow of that energy by means of bleeding, purging, and the minimal intake of food.[2]

Benjamin Rush studied with Cullen at Edinburgh during the 1760s, and he returned to Philadelphia with his medical degree in 1769 as an enthusiastic follower of the Scotsman. But his new beliefs gained him the animosity of the Philadelphia medical establishment, and he later complained that during his first seven years of practice none of his colleagues ever referred a single patient to his office.[3] But by 1790, when virtually all the physicians in the city had accepted Cullen's ideas, Rush himself had come to lose faith in them, and he was attempting to replace them with a coherent new system of his own. First expounded fully in response to the yellow fever epidemic that ravaged the Philadelphia area during the summer of 1793, Rush's new doctrine was ultimately based on Cullen's, but with certain highly significant modifications.

First, Rush rejected Cullen's idea that just as a diminution of nervous energy led to debility, its increase produced the opposite state of spasm. Rush insisted instead that *both* these changes ultimately led to debility. He did so by creating a distinction between two different types of debility— direct and indirect. Direct debility was indeed the effect of a decrease in nervous energy, just as Cullen had claimed; it resulted from what Rush called "an abstraction of usual and natural stimuli." Indirect debility, on the other hand, was what followed an *increase* in nervous energy. It resulted, Rush explained, from "an increase of natural, or . . . the action of preternatural stimuli upon the body."

In other words, unlike Cullen, Rush theorized that a state of debility could be caused by too *much* stimulation as well as by too little. Direct debility might follow from such circumstances as cold, hunger, the excessive loss of bodily matter, or "the debilitating passions of fear, grief, and despair." Indirect debility, on the other hand, could be induced by heat, fatigue, overexertion, or—significantly—by "intemperance in eating or drinking." But whether it was of the direct or the indirect type, Rush argued, debility inevitably left the body in no condition to resist the external forces continually attacking it; and for that reason "debility is always succeeded by increased excitability, or a greater aptitude to be acted on by stimuli." A debilitated individual was predisposed to illness, and the actual "exciting" causes of disease acted on his body "in a manner wholly different from what they do, upon a body in which there is no [such] predisposition."[4]

In Rush's view, then, the immediate stimulus that set off an illness was of less etiological significance than the underlying debility that permitted it to do so. Particular complaints—"those local affections we call pleurisy, angina, phrenitis, internal dropsy of the brain, pulmonary consumption, and inflammation of the liver, stomach, bowels, and limbs"— were "symptoms only" of what Rush called "an original and primary disease." There existed, as he phrased it some years later, "only a single disease, consisting of different forms of morbid excitement, induced by irritants acting upon a previous debility."[5]

Since all illness could be reduced to this single paradigm of debility succeeded by excitement, it followed that the ordinary duty of the physician was to relieve the excitement and thus allow the underlying debility to disappear by itself. In fact, since this underlying debility was itself more commonly "indirect" than "direct"—that is, more often the result of too much stimulation than of too little—it also followed that the very measures which were able to relieve the excitement of the disease would simultaneously alleviate the underlying debility that rendered the body susceptible to excitement in the first place. Because of his doctrine of indirect debility, Rush came to oppose those therapeutic measures that attempted, in accordance with the system of Cullen, to treat certain diseases (specifically, those produced by debility) with stimulants. For the same reason, Rush came to favor measures that promised to soothe and relieve excitement: measures such as reduced diet, controlled regimen, purges, and—especially—bloodletting.[6]

But the doctrine of indirect debility had a significance beyond the immediate therapeutic measures it dictated. In Cullen's system "stimulation" and "debility" were clearly polarized states, with opposite causes and opposite effects. In a certain sense his system was similar to that of the humoralists, even though he dealt in only two elements while they dealt in four, and even though "stimulation" and "debility" were forms of energy while the four humors were palpable substances. The similarity lay in the fact that, for both Cullen and the humoralists, pathological conditions resulted from simple bodily imbalances—imbalances that could be corrected by the addition or removal of one of the body's constituent elements. When Rush introduced the idea that stimulation could itself induce debility, he was implicitly denying that the two states were opposites, and denying as well the idea that disease was the result of a simple imbalance of forces. (Perhaps, like others of his own and succeeding generations, Rush had ceased to perceive the world as sustained by a mercantilist balance of elements.) Rush suggested, even though he never said as much, that stimulation and debilitation were nothing more than different expressions of the same phenomenon, and that it was therefore absurd to think of correcting the one simply by inducing the other. The implications of this shift were highly important for later medical theory.

For all the hostility it initially provoked, Rush's new system eventually came to be just as influential, at least in the Philadelphia area, as his Cullenism had been a generation earlier. The idea that debility could be produced as readily by too much stimulation as by too little, that there was "only a single disease," and that treatment should generally take the form of relieving "excitement," remained in the air even when medical concern shifted, as it did by the 1820s, from fevers to visceral and nervous disorders.[7] Foreign books such as James Johnson's *Essay on Morbid Sensi-*

bility of the Stomach and Bowels and Wilson Philip's *Treatise on Indigestion and its Consequences, called Nervous and Bilious Complaints,* both published in London in 1821, were each reprinted four times in Philadelphia within the following ten years. Both books argued that visceral disorders, because of their effects on the nervous system, were at the root of many ostensibly discrete and unrelated diseases; both argued, furthermore, that these visceral disorders were caused by undue stimulation of the gastrointestinal tract. Neither book was ever published anywhere in the United States other than Philadelphia.[8]

It was in this setting that François J. V. Broussais's *Treatise on Physiology applied to Pathology,* a translation from the French, appeared in Philadelphia in 1826. Although his reputation faded rapidly after 1830 and his name is virtually unknown today, Broussais's theory of "physiological medicine" was widely accepted in France and elsewhere during the 1820s as the long-sought synthesis that had eluded physicians ever since the humoral theory had been discredited two centuries earlier. Broussais's doctrines had been described in this country for the first time in 1821 when the Philadelphia *Journal of Foreign Medical Science,* which had previously reported nothing but Scottish and English work, suddenly began to include a substantial amount of French material. By the middle of the decade, French ideas had been substantially absorbed by the Philadelphia medical profession. In such a context, the translation of Broussais's major work in that city at this time was clearly no accident.[9]

At the heart of Broussais's system lay his acceptance of a doctrine known as "vitalism." According to this doctrine, which had been debated in various forms for several decades, the phenomena that characterized living tissue could not be adequately analyzed by the laws of chemistry and physics. What distinguished animate from inanimate substances was precisely the fact that the laws governing the latter ceased to operate in the former. Living organisms, for instance, resisted such physical principles as the law of gravitation, just as they resisted such chemical principles as the law of decay. The unique process by which living organisms were able to function might be traced, but it could not be explained. As Broussais explained it, some unknown "vital force" acted upon inanimate matter and transformed its natural "chemical affinities" into something he called "organic affinities," which manifested themselves according to a "vital chemistry" that operated according to its own unique laws. This vital chemistry in turn endowed the organism with a number of specific "vital properties."

The most fundamental of Broussais's "vital properties" was "contractility." When living tissue was stimulated by some external force, various kinds of fluid organic matter (blood, for instance) were attracted to it. This process increased the density and volume of the affected area and produced a state of "vital erection," which was characterized by a heightened level of "vital chemistry," including temperature, secretion, and nutrition. Such a vital erection could have one of three consequences: it might subside, leaving a corresponding "diminution of vital phenomena in the affected part"; it might lead to "constriction," by which "the fluids are repelled [in an] organic spasm"; or, it might remain present and induce a pathological state—the state of "inflammation." In the last case, the inflammation would be transmitted to other areas of the organism via the medium of the nervous tissue, "which is especially destined to that use." The degree to which inflammation would spread beyond the spot where it first appeared was a function of the relative abundance of nervous tissue with which the spot was supplied. But, however much it might vary in degree, the sympathetically induced irritation would be identical in kind to the primary irritation: each would cause "the state of life" to be "exaggerated, or rendered more evident."[10]

Since such a pathological process was initially set into motion by the presence of "external bodies" on the surface of internal membranes, Broussais concluded that it was most likely to occur in those two areas of the body most frequently in contact with such external bodies—namely, the pulmonary and the gastrointestinal tracts. These two areas, and especially the latter, were "the most frequently offended of all the parts of the human body by various stimulation, often as abrupt as it is violent." And since the stomach was more abundantly supplied with nervous tissue than any other organ except the brain, it tended to transmit its irritations with greater intensity to other organs. The stomach constituted a complete zone of danger, since it was endowed with a large supply of nervous tissue while at the same time it came into frequent and direct contact with various external agents—food and drink. Moreover, by virtue of its nervous tissue, the stomach was capable of exhibiting a strong sympathetic response to primary irritations located in other areas of the body. For the stomach to become severely irritated, in other words, it was "not always required that a foreign body should be introduced into the digestive passages," since an irritation in any other region could produce the same pathological effect.[11]

For these reasons Broussais believed—and it was this belief that became the trademark of his system—that gastrointestinal irritation was the effective source of virtually all disease, including cancer, syphilis, tuberculosis, and "malignant and pestilential fevers." He denied, as did Benjamin Rush, the existence of any specific diseases. There was in fact only a single disease, and Broussais ascribed particular symptoms—to use Rush's phrase—simply to "different forms of morbid excitement" resulting from that single process: the irritation of gastrointestinal tissue.[12]

If the pathologies of Broussais and Rush had certain basic points in common, their therapeutics were almost indistinguishable. Because disease was produced by inflammation, it had to be treated by a relief of inflammation, and specifically "by a removal of the primary and central gastric irritation." Broussais maintained that the process could best be accomplished by reduced diet and bleeding. (Unlike Rush, who used simple incisions for his "bloodletting," the French physician recommended leeches for this purpose. It was, in fact, Broussais who almost single-handedly caused the importation of leeches to become an important French commercial operation during the 1820s and 1830s.)[13] Broussais denied the efficacy, and even questioned the existence, of what he termed "positive debilitants"—substances that could relieve irritation when taken into the body. For this reason he consistently opposed the use of drugs, which he claimed were merely foreign bodies that would aggravate rather than reduce inflammation. Reduced diet, on the other hand, was effective as a "negative debilitant," which, like bleeding, would reduce inflammation without introducing any foreign substance into the body.[14]

While many of Broussais's positions are obviously the intellectual products of the early nineteenth century, the resemblance between his system and that of Benjamin Rush is nevertheless striking, and it may help account for the flirtation of the Philadelphia medical establishment with "Broussaisism" (as it was called) in the years around 1830. Broussais was able to provide a way of justifying Rush's therapeutics by dressing them in arguments more acceptable to the nineteenth century. The English version of Broussais's *Physiology* was brought out in a second edition in Philadelphia in 1828 and a third in 1832. In addition, two other important works by the same author were published there in 1831 and 1832. With the single exception of a pamphlet on cholera printed in New York during the 1832 epidemic, none of Broussais's work was ever published anywhere in America (or apparently, in the English-speaking world) except Philadelphia.[15]

Sylvester Graham's personal account book records the fact that he purchased Broussais' *Physiology* during his residence in Philadelphia sometime between 1829 and 1831.[16] The account book does not indicate that he ever purchased any works by Broussais's compatriot, Xavier Bichat, but it is no less certain that Bichat accounted for a number of his ideas. It is likely that Graham encountered Bichat by reading Broussais, since the two Frenchmen were born within a year of each other and studied with the same teacher. Broussais began to devise his system only after Bichat's death in 1802 at the age of thirty-one; and "Broussaisism" was generally acknowledged—or at any rate asserted—to be an extension of the discoveries made by Bichat.[17]

Bichat's doctrines, like those of Broussais, stemmed from a vitalistic theory of life. Bichat gave this theory a slight twist, however, which Broussais never picked up but which became a crucial theme in Graham's work. He maintained not only that inanimate and animate matter were governed by different sets of laws, but also that the laws governing animate matter were engaged in a constant struggle to protect the organism against the inanimate laws of physics and chemistry. Everything that surrounds living bodies, Bichat explained, "tends to their destruction," and they would "necessarily soon be destroyed, did they not possess a permanent principle of reaction." Life itself, Bichat suggested, was that principle. Life cannot be "understood" in its nature, but only "measured" in its intensity. The measure of life, he suggested, is "the difference which exists between the effort of external powers" to destroy it, and its own "internal resistance" to that effort. In what are probably his most memorable if not his most significant words—they were memorable at least to Graham—Bichat wrote that "life is the totality of those functions which resist death."[18]

Bichat furthermore proposed, in a distinction that was picked up in different ways by both Broussais and Graham, that an animal body "lives" in two discrete ways at once. On the one hand it lives "internally," or "within itself," and on the other hand it lives "externally," as an "inhabitant of the world." The wholly internal life Bichat termed "organic" (Broussais usually called it "vegetative," since it was the mode of life which animal and vegetable matter had in common); and the external life he termed "animal" (or the life of "relation," as Broussais sometimes called it). Organic functions included respiration, circulation, secretion, and the various digestive functions—all the operations, in other words, by which living creatures assimilated foreign material into their own bodies, and by which they maintained their internal equilibrium.

The animal functions included the five senses along with voluntary motion and intellectuation: the mechanisms by which an animal adapted itself to its environment. (As for reproduction, Bichat argued that it was a special case and belonged, strictly speaking, to neither of the two systems; Broussais included it as an animal function. Sylvester Graham maintained that reproduction belonged to both systems at once, but chiefly to the organic system.)[19] The difference between the two fundamental modes of life, Bichat suggested, was revealed by the condition of sleep, in which animal life was virtually eliminated—the sleeping organism displayed very little sensation, motion, or thought—while organic life proceeded in its usual way. Bichat even argued, from this circumstance, that organic "lives" were twice as long as animal "lives."[20]

Just as Bichat argued that animal life was able to disappear regularly in sleep, he argued similarly that it first appeared only after birth. There was no real animal life in the fetus, whose very movements were "like those of a man asleep." Organic life, on the other hand, was almost fully developed in the fetus. In the same way, animal life ordinarily started to fade well before the diminution of organic life. In fact, to Bichat old age could be defined as the manifestation of the gradual decay of animal life, even while the operations of organic existence might continue to function smoothly.[21] It was clear, in short, that the terms "organic" and "animal" life did not refer merely to two different aspects of the same phenomenon; the distinction between them was real and fundamental. The "organic" and the "animal" systems represented two wholly discrete kinds of life that happened to coexist, continually but not continuously, in every animal organism.

There was a further indication of the disparity Bichat saw between the two modes of life. This was the fact that he believed each of them to be controlled by a separate and functionally independent nervous system. Animal life was directed by a network of nervous tissue focussed in the brain and spinal column. Organic life was directed by a network of nerves, ganglia, and plexuses spread out in and around the different viscera, including the stomach, intestines, liver, and lungs. Unlike the animal nervous system, the organic system lacked any central focus corresponding to the cerebrospinal area. Instead of such a focus, Bichat insisted that each ganglion was "a distinct centre, independent of the others, furnishing or receiving particular nerves as the brain furnishes or receives its own."[22]

In addition to their different structure and function, Bichat maintained that the animal and organic systems were characterized by different properties. All nerves, he noted, possessed both "contractility" and "sensibility,"[23] but he argued that the two systems possessed these properties in different ways. Because the animal system was controlled primarily by the brain, its contractility was subject to the control of the will; and the mere transmission of impulses to the brain, as Broussais wrote, "does not force the will, but merely solicits it, and the percipient centre may resist, and refuse to execute the acts which it demands." The impulses transmitted by the nerves of the organic system, on the other hand, produced "forced movements, which are all in the domain of instinct."[24]

The "sensibility" of the two systems—their capacity to be aware of physical stimuli—differed also, but here the difference was more one of degree than of quality. The animal system possessed sensibility to a far higher degree than the organic system. Bichat illustrated this fact by noting that as the food a person eats passes from the mouth to the stomach— that is, from the animal to the organic realm—the person becomes progressively less aware (or "sensible") of its presence. In only one circumstance was this rule violated, Bichat argued: the organic system assumed a degree of sensibility characteristic of the animal system whenever it became irritated or inflamed. For this reason, the sensory awareness of one's organic life—of the digestive process, for instance—indicated a pathological condition in the organic nervous system. As Broussais wrote, while the organic nervous system "is not sensible in its natural state," it will "become so in a pathological condition, when modified by inflammation," so that "the individual acquires the consciousness of movements, from which he is naturally free in the . . . ordinary state."[25]

Broussais followed, generally speaking, the lead of Bichat. Where the two men diverged, it was generally a result of their different fields of interest—Bichat was, after all, primarily an anatomist and Broussais a pathologist.[26] There were, however, two areas of disagreement between them, and these are worth noting because on each point Graham adopted Broussais's position and not Bichat's. The first issue involved Bichat's denial that there existed any center or focus in the organic nervous system comparable to the brain in the animal system. Bichat denied the existence not only of such a focus, but even of any single "sympathetic nerve" that might serve to link the different viscera into a connected network. In his view the organic system was totally decentralized; each ganglion that composed it was "a distinct centre, independent of the others." What was ordinarily regarded as the "sympathetic nerve" was in fact merely a system of discrete nerves which, taken together, controlled the functions of organic life.

On this point Bichat was at variance not only with successors like Broussais but also with the accepted opinion of his own time. When Bichat was formulating his ideas at the close of the eighteenth century, there was general agreement that the "sympathetic nerve" did indeed exist, but most medical men were inclined to believe its only function was to transmit local sensations and other impulses from one area of the body to another—hence its denomination of "sympathetic." It was precisely such a function that Bichat denied, and it was for this reason that he refused to recognize the "nerve" as a single unit. He insisted, instead, that it was a whole system of nerves with the sole function of directing the operations of organic life. Broussais took another position: He admitted that the "great sympathetic" nerve existed as a single unit, but he insisted that it performed both the function conventionally attributed to it *and* the function granted it by Bichat—that, on the one hand, it sympathetically transmitted impulses from one region of the body to another, and, on the one hand, it regulated the operations of organic life.[27]

It was his belief in the double function of the sympathetic nerve that provided Broussais with the theoretical basis for his doctrine that all disease could be traced to irritation of the gastrointestinal tract, since in his view this tract and the ganglionic network associated with it constituted the single most important arena of organic life. The gastrointestinal tract was the virtual equivalent of the spinal column in the animal system. It was a crucial link in Broussais's chain of "vital laws" that the irritation produced by a local inflammation was sympathetically transmitted to other organs via the nerves of the organic system and "in proportion . . . to the abundance with which an organ is supplied with these nerves." As he noted, the nerves of the organic system are "nowhere . . . so considerable as in the abdominal viscera." By breaking with Bichat over the nature of the sympathetic nerve, Broussais was able to formulate the system of pathology and therapeutics that became known as "Broussaisism."[28]

The second issue on which Broussais disagreed with Bichat, and on which Graham adopted Broussais's position, concerned Bichat's theory that the animal and the organic systems of life were wholly separate and autonomous.

Just as the different ganglia and plexuses of the organic system, and the organs they regulated, were not connected with each other, neither were they connected, in Bichat's view, with the animal system. On this point Broussais was quite explicit in his disagreement. Bichat, he suggested, had encountered "unconquerable difficulties" in trying to draw "a satisfactory line of demarcation" between the two systems—difficulties he would have avoided altogether if he had only recognized that "all the acts of vitality are united and linked together [in] an uninterrupted chain." This connection could be demonstrated, Broussais insisted, on Bichat's own terms—those of anatomical structure. There existed, specifically, a series of "ganglionic cords" that linked the sympathetic nerve "with the nerves of the encephalic domain," and in this way "the cords of the great sympathetic are continuous with the cerebral nerves."[29]

The implications of this connection for Broussais's pathological system are clear: since the two systems of life were interconnected, it followed that "the irritations which are developed in the viscera [are] communicated to the cerebral nerves," and likewise that the irritations "emanating from the brain [are] carried into the ganglionic nerves, and penetrate by means of the latter into the tissues in which these nerves are distributed." In this way there existed a "reciprocity of influence" between the two systems permitting them to serve as "exciters of each other." An irritation of the one would be able to evoke a sympathetic irritation in the other: The entire body formed a continuous and sensitive web of sympathy.[30] This was a resonant notion, and it was not lost on Sylvester Graham as he attempted to formulate a physiological basis for his temperance lectures.

NOTES

1. According to this theory the human body consisted of four different fluids or "humors"—blood, phlegm, and black and yellow bile—each of which contained two of the four fundamental qualities—heat or cold, moisture or dryness. In a state of health, these four humors were maintained in a proper balance; any disruption of this balance would produce a state of disease, the precise nature of which would depend on the nature of the imbalance. Treatment was designed to restore the original balance by adding, in the form of food or medication, any element that might have been lacking, or by removing, through bleeding or purging, any element that might have been present in excess. It is this theory that was at the basis of Luigi Cornaro's dietetics. See Luigi Cornaro, *Discourses on a Sober and Temperate Life*, ed. John Burdell (New York, 1842), pp. 21-23.

2. For a discussion of William Cullen's theories by Rush himself, see Benjamin

Rush, *Autobiography* (Princeton, 1948), p. 80, also Appendix I, pp. 363-364. Actually the most important eighteenth-century theorist of nervous functions was Albrecht von Haller (1708-1777), whose work was of fundamental importance to Cullen.

3. Rush, *Autobiography,* pp. 81-82.

4. Benjamin Rush, *Medical Inquiries and Observations,* 5 vols. (Philadelphia, 1794-98), 4: 123-124, 124-126, 129.

5. Ibid., p. 133. The last phrase is quoted in William B. Walker, "The Health Reform Movement in the United States, 1830-1870" (Ph.D. diss., Johns Hopkins University, 1955).

6. Rush's fondness for blood-letting provoked more hostility than any other of his practices. It eventually led to a lawsuit that became one of the more significant episodes in his career. For Rush's defense of this practice, see "Defence of Blood-letting as a Remedy for certain Diseases," *Medical Inquiries* 4: 181-258. Since Rush's system often was taught in early nineteenth-century medical schools, and his therapeutic practices were generally familiar to physicians, he can be considered highly influential in popularizing the use of calomel (a mercury compound with severe side effects) as a means of "relieving excitement" by purging the digestive tract. Although perhaps less controversial than blood-letting during Rush's lifetime, the extensive use of calomel by American doctors later would become one of the key causes of the attack on regular "allopathic" medicine in the antebellum years. See William Rothstein, *American Physicians in the Nineteenth Century* (Baltimore, 1972), pp. 50-52, 91.

7. An example of this shift is the claim made in 1807 by Thomas Trotter, an English physician, that whereas in the previous 100 years fevers had comprised "two-thirds of the diseases of mankind," by 1800 "nervous disorders" had "taken the place of fevers" and accounted for the same proportion of the diseases "with which civilized society is afflicted." Thomas Trotter, *View of the Nervous Temperament* (London, 1807), p. 13. It is more than probable that it was the idea the medical world held about the nature of disease, not the nature of disease itself, that changed in that 100-year period.

8. James Johnson, *Essay on Morbid Sensibility of the Stomach and Bowels* (London, 1821); Wilson Philip, *Treatise on Indigestion and its Consequences, called Nervous and Bilious Complaints* (London, 1821). Johnson's *Essay* went through its four printings between 1822 and 1831 and Philip's *Treatise* between 1822 and 1825. Other works written by these two men and published in Philadelphia were Johnson's *Influence of Civic Life, sedentary habits and intellectual refinement on human health* (London, 1818; Philadelphia, 1820) and his *Treatise on derangements of the liver, internal organs, and nervous system* (London, 1820; Philadelphia, 1826). Edward Hitchcock included most of these works in the bibliography appended to his *Dyspepsy Forestalled* (Northampton, 1831); and he was especially fond of James Johnson. Johnson himself was strongly influenced by the theories of Bichat and Broussais. While Graham surely read his books—he hardly could have avoided it, they went through so many editions in Philadelphia during his stay there—he took his terminology directly from the two Frenchmen.

9. For an account of the incorporation of French medical doctrines in Phila-

delphia at this time, see Richard H. Shryock, "The Advent of Modern Medicine in Philadelphia, 1800-1850," *Yale Journal of Biology and Medicine* 13 (1941): 728-732. Shryock's article also includes an assessment of the lingering influence in that city of Benjamin Rush. A good illustration of Philadelphia's adherence to vitalist physiology in this period is its resistance to the important discoveries of William Beaumont, the American physician whose experiments helped establish the chemical, non-vitalist view of digestion pioneered by Spallanzani. For details of this episode see J. J. Bylebyl, "William Beaumont, Robley Dunglison, and the 'Philadelphia Physiologists,' " *Journal of the History of Medicine* 25 (1970): 3-21. Not surprisingly, when Graham and other vegetarian theorists felt the need to discount Beaumont's finding that meat was more quickly digested than vegetable matter, they argued that the speed of the *chemical* process involved was in itself a sign of morbid excitement in the *vital* powers that underlay digestion. See James C. Whorton, "Tempest in a Flesh-Pot: The Formulation of a Physiological Rationale for Vegetarianism," *Journal of the History of Medicine* 32 (1977): 129-130.

10. F. J. V. Broussais, *Treatise on Physiology applied to Pathology*, 2nd ed. (Philadelphia, 1828), pp. 42-45.

11. Ibid., pp. xvii-xx.

12. J. D. Rolleston, "F. J. V. Broussais (1772-1832): His Life and Doctrines," *Proceedings of the Royal Society of Medicine* 32 (1939): Part 1, p. 409. For a description and evaluation of Broussais's role in the development of French medicine, see Edwin H. Ackerknecht, *Medicine at the Paris Hospital, 1794-1848* (Baltimore, 1967), chapter 6.

13. Rolleston, "Broussais," p. 411. One historian reports that France imported forty-two million leeches in 1833. Edwin Ackerknecht, *A Short History of Medicine* (New York, 1955), p. 136.

14. Rolleston, "Broussais," p. 409; cf. Rush, *Medical Inquiries and Observations*, 4: 183-186.

15. F. J. V. Broussais's two later books were, respectively; his *Treatise on Chronic Inflammations* (1831) and *Physiological Medicine* (1832). Broussais's reputation declined rapidly in France after 1830 as his theories came under increasingly effective attack. Even in Philadelphia none of his books was published after 1832, presumably because medical opinion in that city kept abreast of current opinion and research. Only someone like Sylvester Graham, who was not a physician, was able to stick for the rest of his life to a position that, while respectable enough when he first encountered it, was soon thoroughly discredited. For an account of the decline of Broussaisism after 1830, see Rolleston, "Broussais," pp. 409-411, and Ackerknecht, *Short History*, pp. 137-138.

16. The account book is referred to in Mildred V. Naylor, "Sylvester Graham, 1794-1851," *Annals of Medical History*, series 3, 4 (1941): 236-240. Since 1941 the account book seems to have disappeared from its repository in the library of the Middlebury Chapter of the Daughters of the American Revolution at Bound Brook, New Jersey.

17. Bichat was in fact a far more important figure in medical history than Broussais, although his significance lay in areas not directly related to his influence on

Graham. Bichat's most important contribution to medical theory was in the field of histology: It was he who first recognized that the bodily organs were not the ultimate units from which the body was constructed—that the organs themselves were constructed of tissues ("membranes," as he called them), and that these tissues actually possessed the qualities previously ascribed to the organs they constituted. The body, Bichat maintained, therefore was composed not of a set of organs but a set of "systems"—cellular, nervous, vascular, glandular, dermoid, epidermoid, and pilious—each of which consisted of a distinct type of organic tissue. In addition, Bichat was the first important representative of the "Paris clinical school" which played a significant role in the development of empirical techniques of medical research.

18. Xavier Bichat, *Physiological Researches upon Life and Death* (Philadelphia, 1809), pp. 1-2. For a suggestive analysis of Bichat's vitalism, see Pedro Lain Entralgo, "Sensualism and Vitalism in Bichat's 'Anatomie Generale,' " *Journal of Medical History* 3 (1948): 47-64. The relationship between Bichat's vitalist theories and those of his predecessors (such as Albrecht von Haller) is discussed in Elizabeth Haigh, "The Roots of the Vitalism of Xavier Bichat," *Bulletin of the History of Medicine* 49 (1975): 72-86.

19. Bichat, *Researches,* pp. 3-4; Broussais, *Physiology,* pp. 524-557; Sylvester Graham, *A Lecture to Young Men, on Chastity, intended also for the Serious consideration of parents and guardians* (Providence, 1834), pp. 42-44. On the other hand, Broussais included the "passions" as a part of animal life, while Bichat placed them in the organic system. Broussais, *Physiology,* pp. 182-219; Bichat, *Researches,* pp. 44-47.

20. Bichat, *Researches,* p. 37.

21. Ibid., pp. 94-134.

22. Xavier Bichat, *General Anatomy, applied to Physiology and Medicine,* 3 vols. (Boston, 1822), 1: 249. Bichat's discussion of the organic nervous system—currently known as the autonomic nervous system—can be found on pp. 249-253.

23. Sir Charles Bell's (1774-1842) important discoveries about the dual structure of nervous filaments, which would have explained anatomically the distinction between these two properties, had not been made when Bichat wrote. They had been made, but not publicized, by the time Broussais wrote his *Physiology.* See Sir Charles Bell, *The Nervous System of the Human Body* (London, 1830).

24. Broussais, *Physiology,* pp. 252-253. See also Pierre Renouard, *History of Medicine from its Origin to the Nineteenth Century* (Philadelphia, 1867), p. 405.

25. Bichat, *Researches,* pp. 70-73; Broussais, *Physiology,* p. 256.

26. When Bichat's work on pathological anatomy was published posthumously in 1825, edited by a disciple of Broussais, it was said that the book proved the two men held identical views. See Xavier Bichat, *Pathological Anatomy. The Last Course of Xavier Bichat, from an autographic manuscript . . .* (Paris, 1825; Philadelphia, 1827). There were some medical men, however, who apparently distrusted Broussais even while they admired Bichat; at least, this is the most likely explanation for the publication of Thomas Henderson, *An Epitome of the*

Physiology, General Anatomy, and Pathology of Bichat (Philadelphia, 1829), an avowed attempt to present Bichat's theories in an unadulterated state.

27. Bichat, *Researches,* pp. 57-62. For a critique of Bichat's views, see Bell, *Nervous System,* pp. 9-10.

28. Broussais, *Physiology,* pp. 44, 249-270, 331-354. For a brief summary of the opinions of both Broussais and Bichat on the nature of the sympathetic nerve, see J. G. C. F. Lobstein, *A Treatise on the Structure, Functions and Diseases of the Human Sympathetic Nerve* (Philadelphia, 1831), pp. 70-72, 76-77.

29. Broussais, *Physiology,* pp. 51-52.

30. Ibid., p. 52.

5. TEMPERANCE

When Sylvester Graham moved to Philadelphia, in June 1830, as an agent of the Pennsylvania Society for Discouraging the Use of Ardent Spirits, that city was at the center of a rapidly burgeoning national temperance movement. As early as the mid-eighteenth century, Philadelphia's large and influential Quaker population had generated much of the earliest American impulse toward humanitarian reform, including the abolition of slavery. It was there that the American temperance movement had been born, nearly half a century before Graham's arrival, and it was there that the movement remained centered until well into the 1830s. The first national temperance convention was held in Philadelphia in 1833. The first temperance tract published in the United States was written by a native of that city, Dr. Benjamin Rush, whose *Inquiry into the Effects of Ardent Spirits on the Human Body and Mind,* first published in 1785 and reprinted many times, remained the standard work on the subject for forty years.

Rush's interest in temperance was consistent with the new medical system he was devising during the 1780s. The effects of liquor on the human body provided him with a perfect illustration of what he meant by "indirect debility." As he noted, "spirits in their first operation are stimulating upon the system," but they come soon afterward to "diminish the action of the vital powers, and thereby produce languor and weakness." Thus debilitated through stimulation, the organism becomes more susceptible to the "morbid excitement" of disease. Rush listed upset stomach, dropsy, jaundice, diabetes, rheumatism, respiratory disorders, epilepsy, insanity, palsy, and apoplexy as the ailments most frequently caused by "the intemperate use of spirits."[1]

But for all the unhappy consequences he attributed to intemperance, Rush's attitude toward drinking was in fact extremely tolerant. He stood in much the same relation to the radical temperance movement of the 1830s as did Luigi Cornaro to the vegetarian movement that was emerging about the same time. What Rush demanded was, quite literally, temperance—not abstinence. He was more concerned about drunkenness than about drinking. In any case, his injunctions applied only to distilled spirits, and not to such fermented drinks as wine, beer, or cider—all three of which he actually recommended as a healthful substitute for hard liquor. As Rush conceded, present custom, past history, "and even nature itself, all seem to demand drinks more grateful and more cordial than simple water."[2]

The first temperance organizations were not formed until early in the nineteenth century. Following Rush's lead, they were designed exclusively to promote moderation in drinking. These earliest societies generally asked their members to pledge that they would not drink excessively, especially during social gatherings. One of the most rigorous of these pledges was drawn up by a temperance group founded in upstate New York in 1808. It demanded that those who signed it promise to abstain from hard liquor except in the event of sickness or on such occasions as public dinners. In at least one instance, a temperance society was actually organized at the local tavern, and after the constitution had been duly signed the members all downed a single shot of hard liquor in order to demonstrate the principles of true moderation.[3]

Even though their scope was extremely limited, temperance societies such as these spread very slowly during the first quarter of the nineteenth century. Not even the churches displayed much interest in the subject. Alcohol was generally served at ministerial ordinations and other ecclesiastical functions. Even in the Puritan period, the New England clergy had accepted alcohol as what one of them, the Reverend Samuel Parris of Salem Village, publicly called "the principle drink that is given to mortal man, being profitable not only to moderate thirst but also to strengthen the heart, and to revive the drooping spirits." (Another Puritan minister, the poet Edward Taylor, occasionally employed alcohol as a metaphor of divine grace. As Taylor once wrote, "It's beer./No nectar like it.")[4]

One of the few clergymen who did become involved in temperance work toward the beginning of the nineteenth century was Lyman Beecher, the Congregational minister at Litchfield, Connecticut. As early as 1812, in a report intended to circulate among his fellow ministers, Beecher recommended a total ban on ardent spirits at ecclesiastical meetings and for general purposes of hospitality, and their partial elimination for regular consumption in families—especially, he argued, in terms which presumably reveal something about early nineteenth-century American dietary habits, its use by young children.

Beecher's interest in temperance increased over the years. Then in 1826, with public concern already beginning to stir in certain areas, he published the first important book on the subject since Benjamin Rush's *Inquiry* had appeared forty-one years earlier. Beecher's *Six Sermons on Intemperance* was more than a new temperance handbook: it helped change the very face of the movement. It repudiated, for the first time, the principle that lay at the root of all existing temperance organizations: that moderate drinking was harmless. "Habitual tippling," Beecher insisted in a remark directed more at the moderation-minded supporters of the movement than at those who opposed or ignored it—"Habitual tippling is worse than periodical drunkenness." It was a serious mistake, Beecher proclaimed, to argue that "the tongue must falter, and the feet must trip" before one was guilty of "criminal intemperance." A person became intemperate the moment that drinking affected his behavior, or even his mood, in the slightest way— by inducing, for instance, a state of "garrulity, or sullen silence; inspiring petulance, or anger, or insipid good humour, and silly conversation."[5]

Beecher based his new definition of intemperance not only on principles of morality but also on "a philosophical analysis of its mechanical effects upon the animal system." In performing this analysis he appealed less to Rush's work than to the kind of European dietary investigations that had been made in the previous twenty years.[6] As Beecher explained, "any stimulus applied stately to the stomach, which raises its muscular tone above the point at which it can be sustained by food and sleep, produces, when it has passed away, debility—a relaxation of the over-worked organ, proportioned to its preter-natural excitement." When frequently repeated, as in the case of regular drinking, this process resulted in "an artificial tone of stomach" that was "entirely above the power of the regular sustenance of nature to sustain." In this way a "vacuum" was created, "which nothing can fill, but the destructive power that made it"—that is, more liquor. When the "protracted use" of drink has widened the gap "between the natural and this artificial tone," and when a man has been drinking for so long a time that "habit has made it a second nature," then no matter how little he may drink on any given occasion "the man is a drunkard" and "irretrievably undone."

Beecher was unequivocal on this score: "Whether his tongue falter or his feet fail him or not, he will die of intemperance." From that point on, a man was no longer master of his actions. "The demand for artificial stimulus to supply the deficiencies of healthful aliment, is like the rage of thirst, and the ravenous demand of famine." Indeed, "it *is* famine: for the artificial excitement has become as essential now to strength and cheerfulness, as simple nutrition once was." Liquor becomes as essential as food, and "nature, taught by habit to require what once she did not need, demands gratification now with a decision inexorable as death, and to most men as irresistible." By this point, the withholding of liquor produces "a living death." But the process of disintegration continues, and "at length, the excitability of nature flags." All the internal organs come to "feel the exhaustion" that has overtaken the body and the mind. At last the drunkard dies from one of the "legion" of diseases "which lie in wait about the path of intemperance."[7]

Six Sermons was published in Boston in 1826, the same year that Graham was ordained as an evangelist in southern Massachusetts. Since Beecher's book was quickly accepted as the battle cry of the temperance movement (or at least of its incipient radical wing), it can be assumed that Graham read it before he left New England in 1827. Yet even though the publication of this book is generally agreed to have marked the great change in the temperance platform from "moderation" to "abstinence," *Sermons* itself hedged noticeably on this very point. Beecher's own fundamental rule of temperance—"THE DAILY USE OF ARDENT SPIRITS, IN ANY FORM, OR IN ANY DEGREE, IS INTEMPERANCE"—was considerably less than a demand for total abstinence: it was only an attack on daily consumption. As Beecher stated elsewhere, "to drink daily, at stated times, any quantity of ardent spirits, is intemperance." In this sense, Beecher's contribution to temperance principles was not so much that he demanded abstinence where others had demanded moderation, but that he condemned the use of liquor in domestic situations as well as for social occasions.

In fact, the very distinction between "intemperance" and "drunkenness" that lay at the heart of the book is by no means as clear as it might appear since Beecher's most powerful argument against moderate drinking was precisely that it led to immoderate drinking. A daily drink, he argued characteristically, may not produce on any given occasion "the intemperance of animal or mental excitement," but it marks "the beginning of a habit, which . . . will not be pursued by one hundred men without producing many drunkards." Dependence on liquor, he noted, is picked up as easily as the plague.[8]

Beecher never claimed that alcohol was in itself harmful to the human body; he claimed that its regular consumption led to a harmful addiction. Even his analysis of the "mechanical effects" of intemperance on the human system is nothing more than a description of how an uncontrollable habit can be created by constant and continued indulgence in a practice that is itself perfectly harmless. The mechanical effects he describes, significantly, are those of "intemperance"—not of alcohol itself. In this context, it is understandable that Beecher conceded (following Rush) that spirits might legitimately be kept in the house "as a medicine."[9] Beecher's attitude toward alcohol was similar to Edward Hitchcock's attitude toward meat: each substance might be dangerous, but each was also necessary. While Beecher did not actually recommend beer and wine as substitutes for hard liquor in the way that Rush did, he nevertheless agreed that "men do not become intemperate on wine," and that beer does "not create untemperate habits."[10]

Because Beecher was concerned more with the formation of addictive habits than with the immediate effects of alcohol on the human body, he did not call unequivocally for total abstinence nor did he in any sense preach what came to be called "teetotalism" (that is, complete abstinence from fermented as well as distilled drinks). Although the first detailed arguments for total abstinence were made as early as 1827 and 1828, it is significant that the first periodical to advocate the practice—the *National Philanthropist,* founded in Boston in 1826 and edited for a time by young William Lloyd Garrison—was printed under the motto, "Temperate Drinking is the down-hill road to drunkenness."[11]

Graham left New England in 1827, at a time when the temperance movement was beginning to experience a sudden surge of popularity. The Pennsylvania Society for Discouraging the Use of Ardent Spirits (later to become the Pennsylvania Temperance Society) was organized in June of that year, partly for the purpose of coordinating the work of the various local socieites that had sprung up in Pennsylvania since the publication of Beecher's *Sermons on Intemperance* the year before. By 1834 there were nearly 150 of these local societies in the state, including thirty in Philadelphia alone. In that same year the thirty-six societies in one county (Washington) reported a membership of 4,813, or one-ninth of the entire population. In addition to the societies there appeared around the state a large number of "temperance stores" and "temperance hotels"—businesses that sold and served no liquor.[12]

Whatever the temperance movement in Pennsylvania may have owed to Lyman Beecher and the example set in New England, it had at least one unique feature—from an early date the medical profession played a dominant role in its activities. In New England, virtually all the leaders of the temperance movement were clergymen such as Beecher or clergymen-educators such as Hitchcock and the Reverend Justin Edwards of the Andover Theological Seminary. But in Pennsylvania many of the leaders were medical men. Temperance in Pennsylvania during the late 1820s was managed by an effective alliance of Presbyterian and Quaker evangelists, and the Philadelphia medical establishment. The medical establishment seems to have dominated the alliance. The second president of the state temperance organization, and eleven of the thirty-six members of its governing board, were physicians; only six were clergymen.[13]

One of the first acts of the newly-formed group was the appointment of a committee of the Philadelphia Medical Society to investigate the relationship between drinking and mortality. The committee studied more than 4,000 deaths in the Philadelphia area and agreed in its report that one-sixth of them were caused, directly or indirectly, by intemperance. When the Philadelphia Medical Society received this report, it formally resolved to use its influence to convince the public to abandon liquor. Sometime around 1830 a group of eighty Philadelphia physicians signed a statement declaring that "men in health are never benefited by the use of spirits," that its consumption is "a frequent cause of disease and death," and that far from being of medicinal value, liquor "often renders such diseases as arise from other causes more difficult of cure and more fatal in the termination." Finally, a "Medical Student's Temperance Society" was formed about the same time at the University of Pennsylvania.[14]

The involvement of so many medical people in the Pennsylvania temperance movement was probably due to the lingering influence of Benjamin Rush, together with the interest in visceral and nervous ailments, and especially the work of Broussais, that characterized medical circles in that state during the 1820s. The involvement of physicians in temperance may help in turn to explain Sylvester Graham's interest in the purely physiological effects of drinking while he was lecturing for the Pennsylvania Society for Discouraging the Use of Ardent Spirits in 1830 and 1831. This connection can be seen with great clarity in the activities of Dr. John Bell (1796-1872), a physician who practiced in Philadelphia and lectured at the Philadelphia Medical Institute (a summer school connected with the University of Pennsylvania).

Bell was an active temperance worker: he belonged to the managerial board of the Pennsylvania Society for Discouraging the Use of Ardent Spirits, and it was he who prepared and read the Anniversary Report submitted to that board in May 1831.[15] Although there is no record of the fact, Bell presumably was a member of the committee of local physicians that had investigated the effect of intemperance on health.

In addition to his temperance work, Bell was one of the two Philadelphia physicians who published the English translation of Broussais's *Physiology applied to Pathology* in 1826. In a preface to the 1828 edition of the work, Bell made no secret of his admiration for Broussais—to whom the translation was dedicated—and for Broussais's predecessor, Bichat. Bell in fact wrote a preface to the translation (in the absence of his co-translator, who was in France at the time) in order to demonstrate that Broussais's system of "physiological medicine" was the logical extension of Bichat's work. Broussais's contribution to medicine, claimed Bell, "consisted in carrying out the ideas of Bichat, and adapting them to the pathology of disease and the practice of medicine."[16]

Bell made it clear that his admiration for Broussais's doctrines was based on something more than their purely scientific merit: "While appealing to nature," he wrote, "they yield the strongest support to sound morality." Although Bell conceded that Broussais himself never drew any moral inferences from his system, he insisted that the doctrines of the French physician demonstrated that there can be "no health for the sensualist—no permanently pleasurable emotions for him who passes the bounds of moderation in the indulgence of his appetites." Only disease and death can result "when the rules of hygiene are neglected, and the laws of sound physiology broken by perpetual stimulation of the gastric surface."[17]

Bell's translation of Broussais's work was first published in 1826, before the temperance movement in Pennsylvania had really come into being. By the time he wrote his preface to the 1828 edition, the movement had burgeoned and the committee of the Philadelphia Medical Society was working on its study of drinking and disease. Possibly Bell's interest in temperance antedated the beginnings of the movement, or even his own discovery of Broussais earlier in the decade. On the other hand, it may have been reading the work of Broussais that disposed him, and other physicians as well, to respond favorably to the popular surge of temperance feeling after 1826. In any case it is clear that, at least for Bell himself, the two circumstances mutually reinforced each other. The doctrines of Broussais provided him with a coherent and convincing pathological basis for his convictions about diet and temperance, and the temperance movement provided him with a means of drawing morally normative inferences from Broussais's system of therapy. Because of Broussais, moreover, he was able to extend his temperance ideas so that they incorporated general principles of diet—food as well as drink—and because of the temperance movement he was able to expand those principles, which Broussais intended only for the sick, into a general regimen for all persons.

This combination of temperance and Broussaisism came to fruition in September 1829, when Bell and D. Francis Condie (another member of the state temperance society's board of managers), with the aid of an "association of physicians," began to publish a biweekly magazine, the *Journal of Health*. The stated purpose of the magazine was "to point out the means of preserving health and preventing disease" by addressing "all classes and both sexes . . . in a style familiar and friendly, and with an avoidance of such professional terms and allusions as would in any way obscure the subject or alarm the most fastidious." The *Journal* was to be mainly filled with the discussion of such topics as "air, food, exercise, the reciprocal action of mind and body, climate and localities, clothing, and the physical education of children."[18] The editors promised in their initial prospectus that "the value of dietetic rules shall be continually enforced and the blessings of temperance dwelt on, with emphasis proportioned to their high importance and deplorable neglect."[19]

Although its contents were, as promised, "devoid of professional terms and allusions"—the *Journal of Health* was in fact the first nontechnical medical magazine published in America[20]—its editors owed an evident debt to François Broussais, Benjamin Rush, and even Jean Jacques Rousseau. They based their temperance position on the existence of a set of "vital or organic laws," wholly distinct from "the laws of inanimate matter," upon which all living things depended for "their integrity of structure and healthy existence." These laws, they affirmed, could "never be infringed without punishment." Digestion was a "vital process" that operated in accordance with these laws and as such it would be "retarded" by drinking distilled spirits, wine, "or even malt liquors." This was the case because alcohol causes "fermentation of the food" in the stomach—replacing the action of vital laws with that of chemical or inorganic laws.[21]

The particular bias of the *Journal of Health* was demonstrated in the opening article of its very first number, which attacked the "popular error" that "nearly all the physical suffering to which the human system is liable" was caused by "weakness or exhaustion." This "fear of debility," the editors claimed, was itself "a fruitful source of improper habits and disease," since it induced anyone who was ill to believe that "all he requires is something to restore strength to his system generally" and thus to take "additional and more stimulating food; some cordial or elixer—some potent tonic!" As a consequence, rather than any permanent improvement, there would occur a "momentary excitement," after which he would become "more and more exhausted; and if he fall not a speedy victim to the disease itself, he too often does to the effects of intemperate habits induced by the remedies to which he has had recourse." Indeed, it was not only in times of disease, but also "during health" that "the same injurious means are resorted to, to sustain the strength of the system." Even "the infant in the nursery is too often pampered into disease, under the ridiculous notion of ministering to its strength." Disease, claimed Bell and Condie, could not be prevented by "the inventions of the cook, the products of the still, or the combinations of the apothecary," but only by "temperance, pure air, exercise, and the subjection of the animal passions."[22]

As for the last of these measures, the *Journal of Health* had little to say except an occasional warning that "the more violent and depressing passions" such as "anger, ambition, jealousy, fear, grief, and despair" tended to "lay the foundation for the most formidable diseases," whereas such "animating affections" as "joy, hope, love, &c." were "highly conducive to health" as long as they were "kept within proper bounds."[23] (It seems clear that the editors did not care to discuss sexual desire among the "animal passions" to be kept under subjection.) About the other measures—especially about temperance, both in drinking and eating—the *Journal of Health* spoke frequently and at length. It maintained that while the body's instinctive dietary needs were altogether trustworthy, these needs were generally perverted by years of training and habit. The perversion of natural appetites would usually begin in infancy itself, when the mother became accustomed to pacifying her wailing baby "by putting it to the breast," even if the real cause of its "infantile uneasiness" had nothing to do with hunger. When the child was weaned, it would be given food "of a mixed and heterogeneous nature" which was "beyond all its real wants." "Its cries are choked now, as in the first stage of its existence, by food." Ordinarily the child would not resist all this feeding, and so "its passively swallowing whatever pap or posset is put into its mouth is mistaken for a real fondness for these substances." Eventually habit would become need, and nature itself would no longer be natural. "We know not under these circumstances how to separate artificial wants from instinctive ones."[24]

For this reason, claimed the *Journal,* it was necessary to establish artificial dietary regulations as a replacement for the instinctive regulations people had lost. Although the magazine did not delineate these regulations in a systematic way, its recommendations proved similar to those in Edward Hitchcock's *Dyspepsy Forestalled*—a book favorably reviewed by the *Journal of Health,* and which afterwards was excerpted in it, along with earlier writers including George Cheyne and Luigi Cornaro.[25] Like Hitchcock, the editors of the *Journal* did not actually recommend the elimination of animal food from human diet, although they came closer than he did to taking such a step, when they asserted that "vegetable substances . . . are fully sufficient of themselves for maintaining a healthy existence."[26]

The magazine took its most radical position on the subject of alcohol. By the middle of 1831, it had come out unequivocally against the use of fermented as well as distilled beverages—the first American publication to do so. To be sure, the *Journal* had not held this position from the beginning. As late as March 1830, it had admitted that malt liquor consumed "in moderation" was "an innocent and wholesome beverage."[27] In May of the next year, however, in an article with the title "Let Us Be Consistent," the editors for the first time pushed the argument beyond the terms in which Lyman Beecher had placed it six years earlier, and insisted that the real issue was not intemperance but alcohol itself. "Alcohol is the denounced poison." Once this point was admitted, it was absurd to justify the use of wine, beer, or cider on the grounds that these drinks rarely led to intemperance. If it was true that fermented beverages contained less alcohol than distilled beverages, it was equally true that they contained "other noxious, and, at times, directly poisonous ingredients" that amply compensated for their relatively smaller amount of "the denounced poison." There was, the editors concluded, only one drink fit for man; and that was water.[28]

Graham began to deliver temperance lectures in the Philadelphia area in mid-1830. In November of that year a notice in a local newspaper reported that he had "astonished and delighted the numerous and crowded audiences which have heard his lectures. Judges, Lawyers, Physicians, and Clergymen as well as the more unlearned," the notice continued, "all degrees of society have listened to him, with equal interest and satisfaction." By the end of November the same paper noted that Graham was lecturing with "truly astonishing" effect to "crowded houses" in the Philadelphia suburbs of Kensington and Northern Liberties—both rapidly industrializing communities that were also being successfully proselytized by evangelical clergymen. Graham seems to have been particularly effective in persuading local factory workers to give up their daily ration of spirits.[29]

Early in December 1830, Graham delivered a series of seven lectures in as many evenings at the German Reformed Church in Northern Liberties.[30] A report on these lectures was printed in the *Journal of Health* on December 8. Brief as it is, this report makes the tenor of the lectures sufficiently clear to indicate the kinds of arguments Graham was employing as early as 1830. To begin with, "availing himself of the aids of chemistry and physiology," Graham argued that ardent spirits were "not called for by the wants of nature," but were "foreign and deleterious principles, which disturb the play of chemical and vital affinities within us." They excite the body temporarily, "only to leave greater weakness than existed before. When they seem to give strength, it is the force of a delirious or maniacal man—violent and irregular, and promptly succeeded by languor and extreme feebleness." While spirits irritated the entire organism, Graham noted that they affected "the stomach first." Large quantities of blood rush there and, in lesser amounts, to the other organs, but there is "no new supply of this vital fluid" available for normal circulatory operations. As a result the entire body begins to misfunction: the skin does not perspire, the muscles cease to contract "regularly and co-ordinately," the gastrointestinal membranes "become inflamed," and the joints are "racked with pains."[31]

While Lyman Beecher had used physiological arguments, among others, in his *Sermons on Intemperance* four years earlier, they were not quite the same arguments Graham employed, nor were they couched in quite the same terms. Beecher had used physiology primarily to demonstrate that alcohol was addictive, and therefore that regular "temperate" drinking led inevitably to intemperance. It was drunkenness that Beecher condemned in the last analysis, and he criticized moderate drinking only because it led to drunkenness. For this reason, the physiological effects he described were simply the creation of an addictive need, a "demand for artificial stimulus" as powerful as "the rage of thirst," a demand "inexorable as death." The physical suffering Beecher described was born exclusively of need and denial. If the life of the drunkard was a hellish one, it was because "the *denial* is a living death."[32]

Graham did not argue in these terms; or, if he did, the *Journal of Health* did not report the fact. His concern was not, apparently, with the addictive properties of alcohol or even with "intemperance" generally, but with the immediate effects of alcohol on the human organism. In other words, he was not interested in its effects on behavior or mood, but on what it did to the normal physiological process. Where Beecher had spoken about the agony of "denial," Graham warned of physiological disruption, "irritation," and pain. To Beecher the most agonizing effect of alcoholic stimulation was that it generated an uncontrollable need for more of the same; to Graham the stimulation itself was the agony.

It was this difference in emphasis that made it possible for Graham to stake out a teetotal position in his early temperance lectures. Beecher could not unequivocally condemn fermented drinks because he admitted that they do "not create intemperate habits." Since Graham was not especially concerned with "intemperate habits," he was able to condemn "every liquid stimulant stronger than water," on the grounds that they were "disturbing to the body, wearing it out sooner, and . . . detrimental to the health."[33]

The emphasis on irritation rather than addiction was a new development in the temperance movement. It is likely that Graham picked it up from someone like John Bell, whom he probably encountered first as a leader in the Philadelphia temperance movement, then as co-editor of the *Journal of Health,* and finally as translator of Broussais's *Physiology Applied to Pathology.* Any doubts on this score should be dispelled by the terminology Graham employed in his lectures—when he claimed, for instance, that liquor contained "foreign and deleterious principles, which disturb the play of chemical and vital affinities within us." It would have been hard for him to speak in this language if he had not read (or at least read about) the works of Bichat and Broussais, and if he had not achieved at least a crude comprehension of the former's vitalism and the latter's theory of pathology. The ideas of these two men formed the basis of Graham's analysis of the physiology of drinking in 1830, just as they would form the basis, two years later, of his analysis of the physiology of epidemic cholera, and, two years later still, of the physiology of sexual desire.

But if French physiological theory provided Graham with the framework for a new and potent set of arguments against drinking, it simultaneously undermined his ability to think of temperance as a separate movement. Once pain and irritation had replaced addiction and drunkenness as the fundamental consequences of drinking, there remained little reason for Graham to limit his argument to alcohol alone, since there existed a variety of other substances which, while less addictive than alcohol, were equally irritating to the gastrointestinal tract. The diversified concerns of the *Journal of Health,* for example, showed how this kind of argument could carry a temperance platform well beyond the confines of the temperance movement and into the more general domain of diet and personal hygiene.[34]

Graham moved in this direction within six months after he had begun to deliver his temperance lectures in Philadelphia. As early as November 8, 1830, it was announced that he would speak on "the health, happiness and long life of Man." The temperance lecture he delivered on December 12 was advertised as "probably his last lecture in this city." But on New Year's Day of 1831, a suburban Philadelphia temperance society announced that Graham would begin a new course of lectures at the Episcopal Church in Northern Liberties. These lecture, to be given three evenings a week, would have as their general subject the relation of temperance to "the organic structure of man." The course.was completed on January 26, when the secretary of the Pennsylvania Society for Discouraging the Use of Ardent Spirits announced that Graham would soon be able to repeat it "in the central part of the city proper, as soon as the necessary arrangements can be made." Apparently there was some difficulty about these arrangements, because Graham seems to have lectured only occasionally during the next four months. The nature of the difficulty can only be surmised, but it is interesting to note that after the end of January, the newspaper notices stopped referring to Graham as an agent of the Pennsylvania Society for Discouraging the Use of Ardent Spirits, and Graham later reported that his connection with the group (like his connection with other organizations before and after this time) had been severed.

Possibly his new position was too extreme for the tastes of the Society.[35] In any case, on May 26, 1831, a new course of lectures—"Mr. Graham's last course for the season"—was advertised to begin four days later at Philadelphia's Franklin Institute, a lecture hall not affiliated with any church. The notice warned that admission would be limited to those with series tickets in order "to prevent too great a crowd, and to secure the same audience throughout the course." This last consideration was something novel, and suggests that Graham had ceased to see himself as an evangelist preaching to whoever might happen to come. It also suggests that he had consciously come to see his temperance message as just a single plank in a much wider platform—a platform too complex to be constructed in a single lecture. The nature of the new subject was revealed in the title he chose to give his new course of lectures—a title he was to employ for the rest of his career as a lecturer, and which he would use eight years later for his two-volume treatise on physiology and hygiene. Graham would lecture, it was announced, on "the Science of Human Life."[36]

NOTES

1. Benjamin Rush, *Medical Inquiries and Observations*, 5 vols. (Philadelphia, 1794-98), 4: 59-61.

2. Ibid., 4: 70-72. In contrasting the deleterious effects of liquor with the beneficial effects of "strong-beer," cider, and wine, Rush insisted that the latter drinks provided the body with "strength, and a power in the system to resist the extremes of heat and cold"; they provided the mind with "cheerfulness, good humour, generosity and social pleasures"; and they improved a person's status in society by providing "friendship, honour, [and] public and private confidence." Quoted *Journal of Health* 1 (1829-30): 265. Rush's principles are summarized in August F. Fehlandt, *A Century of Drink Reform in the United States* (Cincinnati and New York, 1904), pp. 25-30. See also Mason Locke Weems, *The Drunkard's Looking-glass*, 6th ed. (n.p., 1818).

3. Joseph R. Gusfield, *Symbolic Crusade: Status Politics and the American Temperance Movement* (Urbana, Ill., 1963), similarly distinguishes the moderate pre-1830 phase of temperance reform, led by members of traditional local elites in an attempt to maintain control over an increasingly unruly populace, from the more radical post-1830 phase, dominated (as Gusfield sees it) by upwardly-mobile people who used their teetotalism as a badge of middle-class respectability. I would

dispute only the motives Gusfield imputes to the teetotalers. See Chapters 8 and 9 See also Leonard L. Richards, *"Gentlemen of Property and Standing": Anti-Abolition Mobs in Jacksonian America* (New York, 1970).

4. Samuel Parris, "After the Same Manner Also He Took the Cup, A sermon preached in Salem Village, August 6, 1693," in an unpublished sermon book, p. 211, Connecticut Historical Society; Edward Taylor, "Meditation. Cor. 10.4. And all drunk the same spirituall drinke," in Donald E. Stanford, ed., *The Poems of Edward Taylor*, Abridged ed. (New Haven, 1963), p. 181. Parris went on to say that alcohol is "very medicinal, so that being rightly used, by purging the blood, and strengthening the spirits, it prevents many diseases." This is the same language that "Aristotle" used to describe sex.

5. Lyman Beecher, *Six Sermons on Intemperance*, 2nd ed. (Boston, 1828), pp. 9, 11-12.

6. For instance, James Johnson's *Essay on Morbid Sensibility of the Stomach and Bowels* (London, 1821); see also Thomas Trotter, *An Essay, Medical, Philosophical, and Chemical, on Drunkenness, and its Effects on the Human Body*, 2nd ed. (London, 1804; Philadelphia, 1813).

7. Beecher, *Six Sermons*, pp. 12-15.

8. Ibid., pp. 37-39.

9. Ibid., p. 17; also pp. 38-40.

10. Ibid., p. 42. Beecher insisted that while men may not become intemperate on wine, "it is not true that wine will restore the intemperate" (p. 42).

11. Fehlandt, *Drink Reform*, pp. 56-57. It is interesting that the first English temperance organizations displayed a similar reticence on the issues of abstinence from fermented drinks and the use of spirits for medicinal purposes. This correlates with the documented influence of American ideas (especially those of Lyman Beecher) on English temperance reformers. See Brian Harrison, *Drink and the Victorians: The Temperance Question in England, 1815-1872* (Pittsburgh, 1971), pp. 102, 107, and *passim*.

12. Asa E. Martin, "The Temperance Movement in Pennsylvania prior to the Civil War," *Pennsylvania Magazine of History and Biography* 49 (1925): 203. Martin reports that in the city of Chester alone there were forty temperance stores and eight temperance hotels in 1834. (Most of these, it appears, were not new establishments but rather existing businesses that had gone "dry.") See also Othniel Alsop Pendleton, Jr., "The Influence of the Evangelical Churches upon Humanitarian Reform: A Case Study Giving Particular Attention to Philadelphia, 1790-1840," *Journal of the Presbyterian Historical Society* 25 (1947): 15-45.

13. *Poulson's American Daily Advertiser*, March 5, 1831.

14. Harry M. Chalfant, *Father Penn and John Barleycorn* (Harrisburg, 1920), pp. 68-69, 73.

15. *Transactions of the Medical Society of Pennsylvania* 10 (1874): 750; *Poulson's American Daily Advertiser*, May 31, 1831.

16. F. J. V. Broussais, *Treatise on Physiology applied to Pathology*, 2nd. ed. (Philadelphia, 1828), p. viii. But see Thomas Henderson, *An Epitome of the Physiology, General Anatomy, and Pathology of Bichat* (Philadelphia, 1829), preface.

17. Broussais, *Physiology*, p. viii.

18. *Journal of Health*. From the "notice" appended to the end of each number. See, for instance, Vol. 1 (1829-30): 32.

19. *Journal of Health* 1 (1829-30), 1.

20. Frank Luther Mott, *A History of American Magazines, 1741-1850* (New York, 1930), p. 440.

21. *Journal of Health* 1 (1829-30): 41.

22. "Popular Error—Strength and Debility," *Journal of Health* 1 (1829-30): 3-5.

23. "Disordered Passions," Ibid., 1: 164. See also *Journal of Health* 2 (1830-31): 25-26.

24. *Journal of Health* 1: 33-34.

25. Ibid., 1: 5, 203, 229, 311-315; 2: 27-30.

26. "Bread," *Journal of Health* 1 (1829-30): 277; see also pp. 6-7. On the other hand, the same article suggests that "a proper combination of vegetable and animal diet, is the one most friendly to the human constitution, and the best adapted to preserve it in a proper state of health and vigour" (p. 278).

27. "Bread," p. 212. When this article was reprinted in a Philadelphia newspaper that summer, a correspondent wrote in to dispute the statement and to claim instead that water was the only healthful drink for man. *Poulson's American Daily Advertiser,* July 21 and August 31, 1831.

28. *Journal of Health* 2: 272; see also 2: 381. The *Journal's* editors had been extolling the virtues of water since their first number, and they called it "the only fitting drink" as early as August 1830. It was only in May of the following year that the magazine took an avowedly teetotal position. See 1: 209-222; 2: 42-51.

29. For Graham's effectiveness among factory workers, see *Genius of Temperance,* May 4, 1831.

30. *Poulson's American Daily Advertiser,* Nov. 5, 1830; Nov. 27, 1830. The *Genius of Temperance* reported (April 6, 1831) that one of Graham's lectures was attended by "one of the most crowded audiences . . . ever assembled in Philadelphia." See also *The Pennsylvania State Temperance Society Annual Report of the Managers of the Pennsylvania Society for Discouraging the Use of Ardent Spirits* (Philadelphia, 1831), and Othniel A. Pendleton, "The Influence of the Evangelical Churches upon Humanitarian Reform: A Case Study Giving Particular Attention to Philadelphia, 1790-1840," *Journal of the Presbyterian Historical Society* 25 (1947): 30. The best summary of Graham's activities in this period is Edith Cole, "Sylvester Graham, Lecturer on the Science of Human Life: The Rhetoric of a Dietary Reformer" (Ph.D. diss., Indiana University, 1975), 20-24.

31. *Journal of Health* 2: 113-114.

32. Beecher, *Six Sermons on Intemperance.* The italics added.

33. *Journal of Health* 2: 114. It should be remembered that this report on Graham's lecture was printed some five months before the *Journal's* own editorial conversion to teetotalism.

34. The same thing is true, of course, of such books as Edward Hitchcock's *Dyspepsy Forestalled* (Northampton, 1831). But even here there is a difference, and an instructive one. Around 1830 Hitchcock's views paralleled Graham's; all he lacked was an acquaintance with French physiology—a fact evident from his bibliography. For that reason he was unable to go either teetotal or vegetarian.

35. The Society did not adopt a teetotal position until 1834, by which time such a position was considerably more common than it had been in 1830. When the group did go teetotal, its name was changed to the Pennsylvania Temperance Society. The change of position was accompanied, incidentally, by the resignation of the president of the Society—an obvious indication that teetotalism did not please all temperance people even at that time. After the *Journal of Health* shifted to teetotalism in 1831, one of its favorite targets became "the rich man of a Temperance Society" who "is allowed to drink wine, which contains from 20 to 30% of alcohol," while he condemns the poor man who drinks liquor which contains "from 40 to 50% of alcohol." *Journal of Health* 2: 114. The teetotaler's disapproval of the wine drinker is comparable to Lyman Beecher's earlier displeasure toward the "habitual tippler." Graham reports the conclusion of his association with the organization in his *Lectures on the Science of Human Life,* 2 vols. (Boston, 1839): 1: vi.

36. *Poulson's American Daily Advertiser,* Nov. 8 and Dec. 10, 1830; Jan. 24, Jan. 29, Feb. 1, Mar. 18, May 7, May 26, 1831. Mildred Naylor, working from Graham's unpublished account book, claims that "within nine months [of his engagement by the Pennsylvania Temperance Society] he was delivering lectures on 'Chastity,' 'Courtship and Marriage,' 'The Intellectual and Moral Faculties,' 'The Prevention and Treatment of Cholera,' 'Diet Reform,' etc." No report survives on Graham's first series of lectures on "The Science of Human Life." Mildred V. Naylor, "Sylvester Graham, 1794-1851," *Annals of Medical History* 4 (1941): 236-240.

6. CHOLERA: AN EPIDEMIC OF DEBILITY

Sylvester Graham left Philadelphia in June 1831, to visit New York City. He had received an "urgent invitation" from William Goodell, editor of the *Genius of Temperance*, who had heard Graham and sensed that he possessed the "rare talent of interesting all who hear him." Goodell suggested in the columns of his newspaper (formerly edited under another title by the young William Lloyd Garrison) that a "commercial emporium" such as New York was especially needful of a man with Graham's engaging oratorical ability and his commitment to true temperance principles. After Graham delivered a heavily-promoted series of lectures in New York's Clinton Hall, he returned to the Philadelphia area for the summer. There he gave his lecture series several more times and attended the state temperance convention in Harrisburg before leaving once again for New York City in November. The two series of lectures he delivered there that winter (one at Clinton Hall and the other at the Mulberry Street Baptist Church) were so successful that each had to be repeated to overflowing crowds.[1]

Graham was still in New York in March 1832 when dread news arrived that was soon to propel him into something approaching national prominence. A lethal epidemic of cholera, spreading out of Asia, had passed through Europe and was now expected to reach the North American continent within a few months. In anticipation of its arrival, conflicting analyses of the nature of the disease, and conflicting recommendations about how it might be prevented (or, if it struck, how it might be treated), began to appear in newspapers, books, and even sermons. In its own way, cholera became as intense a subject of national debate in 1832 as the National Bank. The years 1832 and 1833 saw the publication of literally hundreds of occasional pieces on the subject, written from a variety of conflicting medical, moral, and theological positions. Many of the works advised the American people to fortify themselves against the approaching epidemic by adopting a hearty, stimulating diet of meat, spices, and brandy. But other writers set forth precisely the opposite set of recommendations. Among the latter was a report prepared by the Philadelphia College of Physicians for the municipal Board of Health of that city, a report authored by John Bell, editor of the *Journal of Health*.[2]

Graham was lecturing in New York on the "Science of Human Life" as the epidemic approached. In March 1832, at the conclusion of one of his lecture courses, he announced that he would deliver an additional talk about the dreaded disease—its nature, prevention, and proper treatment. His lecture, at the Baptist meeting house, was attended by more than 2,000 people, and when the epidemic finally arrived in the United States in June, Graham was asked to repeat the talk. He first spoke in New York City towards the end of that month, again in July at Albany, and later in the year in New Bedford, Fall River, and Providence—the same area of southeastern New England in which he had been ordained as an evangelist six years earlier. In each city, Graham's lecture provoked a combination of fervent support and hostile ridicule. (One New York City newspaper called it a "masterly performance," while another warned that "if the cholera comes here, all the Grahamites will certainly die.")[3]

Such a mixed reaction is easy to understand. While Graham's general opinion about the nature of cholera was by no means unusual—he was, after all, not the only man in the country to have been influenced by François Broussais—his preventive and therapeutic recommendations were considerably more extreme than those of other exponents of French physiology such as John Bell and Francis Condie, who at least did not deny, as Graham did, the efficacy of opium and other artificial preparations in the treatment of the disease.[4] In any case, with the delivery of this lecture around the Northeast, and its publication in expanded form the following year, Sylvester Graham achieved a measure of fame and notoriety. He also gained a sizable following that provided scores of testimonials to the success of his system of diet and regimen—first of all in protecting those people who adopted it from the effects of the epidemic, and afterwards in restoring the general health and vitality of those who had theretofore been chronically ill.[5]

It must have been evident to Graham's audiences that if his analysis of cholera was correct, it led to a view of health and disease extending far beyond the emergency measures that might have to be taken in response to an occasional epidemic. Graham made no attempt to conceal the fact that the lecture was simply a specific application of the principles of the science of human life. All that he did conceal (and this was a deception he kept up for the rest of his career) was the origin of those principles in the writings of Benjamin Rush, Xavier Bichat, and Broussais.

Broussais himself actually wrote an essay on cholera that was translated into English and published in New York at the time of the epidemic.[6] The resemblance between Broussais's analysis and Graham's did not go altogether unnoticed in the controversy over the latter's recommendations, and Graham was accused on at least one occasion of having copied his ideas from Broussais's essay. Graham expressed surprise at any resemblance, and insisted he "had read no other medical treatise on the cholera whatsoever" when he composed his own lecture. In fact, he claimed, his knowledge of the disease had been gleaned solely from newspaper accounts of the epidemic's progress through Asia and Europe. He had formulated his analysis exclusively by applying to these accounts what he knew to be "the true principles of physiological and pathological science."[7]

However misleading this disclaimer may have been, it was, in all probability, true: Graham did not need to be acquainted with this particular essay of Broussais in order to utilize a conceptual framework in which he was already well-versed. It was true that nowhere in the *Lecture on Cholera* (or, for that matter, anywhere else in his writings) did Graham mention the names of Broussais, Bichat, or Rush. But to anyone acquainted with contemporary French physiology, the source of his "true principles" would have been clear enough. Indeed, he all but proclaimed it on the very first page of his lecture: "Life," he announced—and while he did not identify the author of this statement he did enclose it within quotation marks —" 'Life is a temporary victory over the causes which induce death.' "[8]

It was not simply this motto, however, that Graham owed to Bichat or Broussais. The first twelve pages of the *Lecture*, in which cholera was not once mentioned, simply expounded his own amalgam of the major principles of the two Frenchmen. At the core of Graham's vision lay Bichat's brand of vitalism, with its peculiar emphasis on life as a constant battle between opposing forces. Graham defined life (and this time the words were his own) as a "continued antagonistic conflict between vitality and the more primitive affinities of inorganic chemistry":

In producing each and all of its peculiar and legitimate results, vitality necessarily overcomes the laws, and counteracts the affinities of inorganic matter; and exerts molecular affinities, of a totally distinct and opposite character,—which result in aggregations and structures, entirely different from those of inorganic matter:—and hence it is true, that all the inorganic affinities in Nature, are averse to organic structure, and life: and hence also, it is true, that life maintains its power, and performs its functions, in opposition to the ordinary laws of inorganic matter, and within its own appropriate domain, resists the operation of those laws, while its power is paramount.[9]

Following both Bichat and Broussais, Graham distinguished between animal and organic life, the former comprising the "organs and powers of sensation, voluntary motion, and volition," and the latter the "organs and powers concerned in the grand function of nutrition: such as appertain to digestion, respiration, circulation, secretion, absorption, excretion, etc." Each of these lives, he went on, was controlled by a separate network of nerves: those pertaining to animal life "are connected with the brain and spinal marrow, and are distributed principally to the muscles of voluntary motion, and to the sensitive surface of the body, or external skin," while those pertaining to organic life "are believed to originate with the organs themselves, in a kind of rudimentary brain, or bulbous enlargement of nervous substance, which is called a ganglion or knot, of which there is a large number in the different parts of the body."

It was, naturally, the organic system that was Graham's chief concern, and he described it in considerable detail. He noted how the ganglia, or areas of enlarged organic nervous tissue, threw off a variety of "cords or branches." Some of these branches, he explained, connect directly with each other and form a "general union or system of the whole"—in other words, a sympathetic network—while others connect via the brain and spinal column with the animal system of nerves; and still others "interweave and inosculate" with themselves to form "plexuses," or large masses of nervous matter, which in turn reach out "to supply the stomach, and heart and lungs, and liver and kidneys, and all the other organs concerned in the general function of nutrition."

Two of the largest ganglia, the "semilunar" ganglia, branch out to form the *solar plexus,* a large body of nervous tissue located in front of the spine, which "constitutes a kind of common center of action and sympathy, to the whole system of organic nerves." The *solar plexus* achieves such importance by giving off branches "in every direction, to enter into other plexuses, and to supply organs." In this way, Graham concluded, "all the nerves of organic life are intimately woven together into a common web of sympathy, and harmony of action—pervading all the organs concerned in the general function of nutrition; bringing them into general and special relations, and supplying them with that peculiar vital power by which each is enabled to perform its particular office."[10]

Graham's concept of animal and organic life, like his vitalism, was derived from both Bichat and Broussais, but it is significant that just as his vitalism took the distinct tone of the former, so his peculiar emphasis on the primacy of organic life was characteristic only of the latter.[11] For Graham, as for Broussais, it was the organic nervous system alone, by virtue of its exclusive control over what Graham called "the grand vital function of Nutrition," which maintained the powers of vitality in a living organism and which therefore prevented it from falling under the government of "inorganic affinities" (i.e., death). "It is by the power derived from or through these nerves," Graham wrote, "that the food is transformed into chyme, and the chyme into chyle, and the chyle into blood." The organism can survive only by converting foreign matter "into its own substance," and without the "living stomach," food would "gradually take on a chemical action, and soon run into fermentation and putrefaction, and pass entirely into other forms of inorganic matter." Since it is the system of organic nerves which supplies the energy that alone can overcome this natural tendency, it is literally true to say that "the vital power which resists, counteracts, and subdues, chemical affinities and noxious agents—the vital power which maintains its victory over the causes which induce death, resides in or acts through, the nerves of organic life."[12]

Both its physiological function and its anatomical structure, then, pointed to the importance of the gastrointestinal tract. As the focal region of organic existence, that system played the key role in insuring the maintenance of life. The gastrointestinal tract was integrally connected, moreover, with every other part of the body: The entire lining of the alimentary canal, from the mouth to the anus, is "one sheet of sympathy." This was especially the case with the lining of the stomach, which was "peculiarly the center of sympathy to the whole organization." Supplied as it was with nerves from the *solar plexus* and the *medulla*

oblongata, the stomach is thereby "brought into distinct and special relations with the brain, heart, lungs, liver, skin, and indeed with all the
organs of the system." Consequently, "every affection and every disturbance of the stomach influences, in a greater or less degree, every
organ and every function of the body." When the stomach functions
properly, "all the vital functions of organic life are most vigorously and
perfectly performed." But when the stomach becomes disordered, then
"every other organ in the system sympathizes, and every other system
languishes."[13]

Still expounding the doctrines of Broussais and Bichat, Graham noted
that healthy people are not ordinarily aware of the organic processes (such
as digestion) that continuously take place within their bodies. This absence
of consciousness was due to the fact that "in their healthy state, the nerves
of organic life have no sensibility." But these nerves, Graham continued,
"are capable of being irritated into a state of excessive irritability," and
whenever such "preternatural and diseased excitability" exists, it is impossible for the internal organs to maintain a "healthy performance."
Since the stomach is the sympathetic center of the body—"a kind of retina
or sensorium to the nerves of organic life"—it followed that a diseased
stomach "cannot suffer alone," but quickly spreads its irritation to the
whole system of organic nerves, and through them to the organs they supply. The condition of these organs thus invariably corresponds to "the
general condition of the digestive apparatus, and especially the stomach."[14]

In a state of general irritation, the body becomes debilitated and—shades
of Benjamin Rush—susceptible to "the action of morborific causes." Moreover, such an irritation inevitably drains "the vital energies of the tissues,"
and thereby "impairs those natural and peculiar sensibilities, which constitutionally adapt the tissues to their natural and appropriate stimuli."
Not only does irritation cause pain, in other words, but by diminishing the
supply of vital energy it renders the various organs incapable of responding
to the very stimuli upon which their normal operation depends. The digestive organs, for example, lose their ability to respond to the presence of
food. Suffering at once from irritation and debility, the body loses its
ability to transform foreign matter into its own substance and to maintain
its own organic affinities; and if the process is not reversed, the ultimate
result is "disorganization and death."[15]

It was irritation, then, and particularly irritation of the stomach, upon
which Graham placed the primary responsibility for disease. Up to this

point, he was speaking simply as the disciple of Broussais. But it was precisely here that the temperance campaigner and social critic began to emerge from behind the neutral terminology of the physiological theorist. In the process it became apparent to what extent the temperance movement had become associated, in Graham's mind, with a general critique of life in Jacksonian America. The human body, with its complex system of organic nerves "integrally woven together into a common web of sympathy, and harmony of action," to Graham had become the sensitive register of social change. "Almost every circumstance and influence in civic life," he lamented, was leading to "preternatural irritability and diseased sensibility"—to "undue excitements and exercises of the mind, and of the passions." These unsettling influences—and the list of them formed a litany that Graham would repeat without significant variation for the rest of the decade—included what he referred to as "the various customs and circumstances of artificial life": all the "debilitating" developments of modern housing, dress, transportation, and, of course, diet.[16]

Diet posed the most serious threat. Because the digestive system was the vital center of organic existence, violations of its "constitutional" laws would inevitably destroy the tenuous "harmony of action" that was necessary to sustain health, and life itself.

> Worst of all, the habitual use of artificial stimulants, such as the heating and irritating condiments of the table, and more particularly the various narcotic and alcoholic substances;—all act upon the stomach to disturb its functions, and to impair the health of its nervous and muscular tissues, and consequently, tend to debilitate that organ, and by continued or repeated irritation, to develope [sic] and establish in it a diseased excitability and irritability, resulting often in chronic or acute inflammation, and painful sensibility and disorganization.[17]

So severe were the effects of these practices, according to Graham, that they would actually kill on the spot were it not for the fact that the practices themselves were ordinarily "entered into by very small degrees of increase." Only the gradual quality of the initiation, Graham argued (in much the way Rousseau had argued in *Emile*), insured that its consequences would not be acute, and ultimately so perverted the instincts as to render the practices pleasurable. For instance, if a non-initiate were suddenly to chew a large quantity of tobacco—"that most loathsome of all sub-

stances, one of the most powerful narcotic poisons in the vegetable kingdom"—there would be no doubt that "the natural susceptibilities of his
nerves would give the alarm instantly." Within a short time the "distressing sympathy" that ensued would extend to the stomach and the brain,
and finally to the entire system. "All the energy of vital resistance would
be summoned up": vomiting and other violent reactions would result as
the system attempted to "reject the destructive poison." In the end, "if
the vital powers were sufficient to sustain the conflict," then "the individual would survive; if not, the most distressing exhaustion, and collapse, and death would ensure." Witnessing such a situation, nobody could
deny the "deleterious properties" of tobacco. But it was surely no less
harmful simply because people did not generally partake of it—or alcohol,
or any "narcotic"—in quantities sufficient to produce this kind of trauma.
Indeed, the ultimate harm was, if anything, greater when the initial dosage
was a small one continually repeated over a period of time, since in that
case the system would cease to respond by attempting to expel the poison,
and, ultimately, would become dependent on it even for its ordinary
stimulation.[18]

In such a state of dependence, according to Graham's theory, the jaded
system would lose its "natural" sensibility to external stimuli, and its
powers of resistance against the omnipresent sources of disease would be
correspondingly diminished. While these sources were to be found everywhere, it was only to an organism that was already in a state of debility
that they presented any real danger. But dependence on the stimulating
forces present in the modern world had, in fact, debilitated the greater
part of humanity in just such a way. For that reason, Graham concluded,
it should not be a "cause of wonder" that so many people were afflicted
with a variety of "chronic and acute diseases," or that any number of
"seemingly trivial causes" should manage to "superinduce an endemic or
epidemic disease." The truth of the matter, Graham insisted, was that
both the incidence and the severity of any disease "corresponds with the
reduced state of the vital power of resistance in man"; and considering the
extent of human dependence on "artificial stimulants," such resistance is
dangerously low. Indeed, it seemed to Graham as if most Americans were
actually conducting a deliberate experiment in brinksmanship—"to ascertain
how near they can run to the line of death, and still maintain life!"[19]

It was in this context that Graham considered the cholera epidemic of
1832. When a healthy gastrointestinal tract becomes irritated, the body

tries to relieve the irritation by means of "a mild form of diarrhoea," and under ordinary circumstances this natural action is sufficient therapy. It was precisely this normal physiological response to gastrointestinal irritation that constituted, in its nonepidemic form, what was generally known as *cholera morbus,* or "spasmodic cholera." The very symptoms of the disease—vomiting and diarrhoea—resembled those of the man who chews a large dose of tobacco for the first time. The similarity was no accident, for cholera, too, was nothing but the body's attempt to purge itself of poisonous impurities—it was "the constitutional means, by which the system instinctively expels offensive and disturbing substances from the alimentary canal."[20]

In itself, then, cholera was not necessarily a dangerous disease. In fact, it was "far from being alarming, unless the disturbing cause is intrinsically and fatally poisonous"—unless, in other words, the original irritation happened to be produced by a lethal substance. But that was only rarely the case since the irritating substance was usually quite harmless. The real danger thus lay neither in the "disturbing cause" nor in the body's symptomatic reaction to it, but in the general condition of the body at the time of its disturbance. Cholera was fatal only when the organic nervous system had been so seriously impaired by prolonged exposure to artificial stimulation that it was incapable of responding in a natural way when beset by irritation. Under such conditions vomiting and diarrhoea, instead of relieving the irritation, served only to increase it. "A morbid irritation once fully induced, in such a system, will not subside even when the first exciting cause is removed; but feeds and increases itself by its own action."

The increased irritation in turn aggravated the vomiting and the diarrhoea, and the ensuing vicious cycle was often terminated only by death. Such a pathological reaction took place whenever the already debilitated gastrointestinal tract was irritated. It established itself as an "abnormal centre of action" in the body, attracting to itself both bodily fluids and vital energy. The original irritation, "excited to madness by the acrid fluids which are pouring in from every corner, and producing an excitement which distracts the normal distribution of nervous energy, from the natural centers to the several [affected] organs . . . blindly drags all the vital energies into the vortex of its own maniacal fury."[21]

It was only because the American people were "strongly disposed to disease, of any and every kind," then, that so many of them were falling prey to cholera. In view of their habits, Graham argued, such a result was only to be expected. "Innumerable as are the irritating and debilitating causes which are continually disturbing and impairing the organic function, and diminishing the vital power of resistance, can it be a matter either of sympathy or surprise that a highly morbid irritability of the stomach and intestines, should obtain in a very large portion of the human race?" Since so many people were in this vulnerable condition, it took very little to push them over the brink and induce in them the severest forms of the epidemic of 1832.

An adscititious [i.e., nonessential] cause, which would scarcely affect, in any degree, a healthy system, may now be sufficient to induce the most violent and fatal disorder. In such a state of things, sudden atmospheric changes, or the presence of noxious gases or effluvia—together with exposures,—fatigue,—exhaustion,—improper kinds, quantities or conditions of food,—free use of heating and irritating condiments—fear—anger—veneral excess—and above all, excesses in alcoholic and narcotic substances, acting directly upon a morbidly susceptible and irritable stomach, and through it on the whole system, the utmost disorder must necessarily ensue.[22]

Graham even suggested that it was not always necessary for there to be any extrinsic or "adscititious" cause at all. It was possible, under some circumstances, for the human system itself to provide a catalyst that would induce an attack of cholera. When a person is already susceptible to the disease, it may sometimes take nothing more than a state of mind—fear, perhaps (for example, the very fear of contracting the disease)—to produce "every symptom and effect" of cholera, including death itself. "In certain conditions of the body, mental action [alone] may so affect the nerves of organic life, as to cause that gastrointestinal irritation, which is the basis of all the symptoms of spasmodic cholera." That it was possible for "certain actions of the mind" to induce "certain conditions of the nervous system" was amply demonstrated—and in the early 1830s this surely must have been a resonant analogy—by the "involuntary spasms" that so frequently affected those in attendance at revival meetings.[23]

Only in this limited sense, argued Graham, was it correct to speak of the present outbreak of cholera throughout the world as an "epidemic." In the ordinary sense of the word, the disease was not even contagious. Its rapid progress from Asia through Europe to America could be seen simply as the result of panic operating upon a series of populations whose generally intemperate habits had debilitated their bodies steadily over the years. In any case, the disease was not caused simply by coming into contact with a person who suffered from it. Indeed, Graham insisted, "I do not believe that any disease to which the human body has ever been subject is *absolutely* contagious." That is to say, since no disease ever comes about entirely by virtue of extrinsic causes but at least to some extent through the action of the human body itself—"by the violation of those laws of life which appertain to the highest state of human welfare"— it follows that no disease is contagious except to those persons whose "general predicament of vital condition and sensibility" is imperfect.

Different diseases in effect become contagious at different levels of prior susceptibility, but no disease is contagious to an individual whose organic health is perfect. Consequently, Graham argued, "the human constitution is still capable of being elevated above the susceptibility to any contagious disease." In any particular instance the question of whether an individual will or will not succumb to an "epidemic" can be answered only by reference to "the condition of his body." That condition, he concluded, "depends very much, if not entirely, on his own voluntary conduct."[24]

In Graham's view, then, the cholera epidemic was essentially, even in the physiological sense, a symbolic event. The disease itself was nothing; what made it lethal and epidemic were the "customs and circumstances of artificial life" that had reached so deep as to subvert the most basic structure of human need and behavior. The epidemic was the manifest expression of all those forces that had transformed the world, and the people who inhabited it, from a source of vibrant resilience and inner serenity into an arena of irritation, disorder, and fevered, destructive energy. Gnawing at the vital core of the human spirit, relentlessly penetrating hitherto-unbreachable geographic barriers, cholera was an apt symbol of the extent to which Americans had lost their self-sufficiency and become vulnerable to a new set of potent and seemingly incomprehensible forces. In 1832 Sylvester Graham used the cholera epidemic, as Andrew Jackson that same year used the Second National Bank, as a resonant symbol of everything that had gone wrong with the nineteenth century.

It was not an altogether irrational connection. Recent scholarship has revealed that the epidemic of 1832, transmitted exclusively by personal contact, was generally limited in its effects to urban or commercial areas—and, in fact, that the paths along which it spread were also the most important marketplace routes. Cholera entered the country at its largest port, New York City. From there it spread across the nation via two major avenues: one course went up the Hudson River Valley and along the Erie Canal to western New York, then down the Ohio Canal to the Ohio and Mississippi Rivers; the other main route went northward and southward from New York City along the Atlantic Coast. In a very real sense, then, the cholera outbreak—the first national epidemic in American history—was a creature of the marketplace economy.[25]

Graham obviously sensed the presence of this connection, but he was able to articulate its nature only in a shadowy and an ultimately misleading fashion. Recognizing that the cholera epidemic was more than a random event—that it was somehow connected with "the customs and circumstances of artificial life"—he was able to explain the enigmatic pattern of its devastation only by recourse to a great and characteristic Jacksonian evasion: the "voluntary conduct" of individuals.

From such a position, it followed that prevention was more practical than cure. In Graham's view, prevention meant insuring the health of the organic system through the radical regulation of diet and regimen. It was on this point that the *Lecture on Cholera* aroused the greatest controversy. Most people mistakenly believed, reported Graham, that the most effective precaution they could take against the epidemic was to avoid debility at all costs: to adopt "a generous system of diet," including the free use of animal food, wine, and brandy. There was, he argued, no error more dangerous than this. While it was true that a reduced diet might create a temporary state of animal weakness, or "muscular debility," such weakness was altogether different from that dangerous "functional debility" of the organic system which rendered the body susceptible to disease. Indeed, it was often the case that "the very means by which we diminish the muscular power of the voluntary organs, increases the vital powers in the nerves of organic life." Weakening the animal system (that is, the muscles), in other words, might actually strengthen the organic system. Since cholera was a disease whose effects were limited exclusively to organic life,[26] even the muscular weakness that might initially accompany a reduced diet, far from increasing one's susceptibility to cholera, could itself help to prevent the disease.[27]

On the contrary, it was crucial to avoid any items "calculated to irritate, and debilitate, and inflame the alimentary canal." Most conspicuous in this category were substances that provided only stimulation and lacked any nutritional value. The list included alcohol in all its forms, tobacco, opium, and spices such as mustard, pepper, and even salt—all of which were to be "entirely avoided, with the most rigid and inflexible scrupulosity." (Graham noted that the epidemic had taken a far higher toll in Paris than it had in London, and he attributed this difference, in part, to the fact that the temperance movement had begun to flourish in the latter city shortly before the epidemic struck, whereas in Paris the city officials were publicly recommending brandy as a preventive measure.) Only slightly less dangerous were such stimulants as tea and coffee, both of which were "decidedly pernicious to health," and which, if they could not be avoided altogether, were to be indulged in "very sparingly."[28]

At the opposite extreme, habitual indulgence in those foods—never "natural" ones—that consisted of pure or almost pure nutriment, with no admixture of non-nutritious and non-irritating bulk, might be equally harmful. Whenever the nutritious properties of food were separated "by artificial means" and eaten in "concentrated form," the alimentary tract became weakened as a result of the effort involved in digesting so much nutritious matter. To be truly healthy it was necessary for food to contain a due proportion of both nutriment and bulk. Therefore, it was imperative that people avoid the concentrated form of all foods, even those which might be perfectly healthful in their natural and unconcentrated state. Soups of all kinds, as well as artificial preparations such as cream and butter, were thus to be shunned. Above all, however, it was white bread—bread made from granulated "superfine flour," from which the bran, or non-nutritious bulk, had been artificially removed—that fell into the category of concentrated food, and for which Graham reserved particular venom. Even the healthiest person in the world, he insisted, "could not very long survive" on a diet of "the very best superfine flour bread and water."[29]

What one could survive on very well, and what Graham recommended enthusiastically as the ideal food, was the recipe that soon became associated with his name—bread made from "good unbolted wheat meal, coarsely ground," and served (to insure that the heat of cooking had ample time to dissipate) "when at least twelve hours old." Graham wrote, "There is no article of artificially prepared food known in civic life, the use of which more invigorates the alimentary canal, and restores, and keeps up the regular and healthful functions of the stomach and intestines." There was, in fact, no food more nutritious, more therapeutic, or more "easy to digest" than bread made from unbolted flour. It was one of the few foods that was safe and beneficial at all times and under all circumstances, even though farinaceous substances, such as "plain, boiled rice" and "coarse, Indian hominy" were almost as good.[30]

As for meat, it was to be regarded with the utmost caution. People would be safest if they abstained from it altogether; if they could not, they should limit themselves "to a little boiled or roasted beef or mutton once a day, without any made gravy, and without any seasoning." In 1832 Graham was still hedging on the vegetarian question. There was little doubt where his own feelings lay, but he seemed uncertain as to how far he could go in making them an obligatory part of his system. He ended up with an ambiguous statement, relying on the epidemic to provide himself with a convenient cover.

> A plain, simple, nourishing vegetable diet is decidedly most conducive to permanent health and longevity. It is less stimulating, and therefore does not wear out the susceptibilities and energies of the living tissue so rapidly, nor does it tend so powerfully to produce chronic and acute disease of any kind, as a free use of animal food. Hence it is in all respects a safer diet, during the prevalence of malignant and epidemic diseases.[31]

But however faithfully a person might adhere to it, a vegetable diet was not alone sufficient to insure good health. Graham continually explained that diet was only one of two crucial areas of potential danger: the other was sexuality. It was, for example, in India that the present cholera epidemic originated, Graham observed, and the population of that country was known to consume little if any animal food. But while the Indians were indeed vegetarians, in Graham's opinion they were not "temperate," either in their dietary or their sexual practices. First, their diet was extremely bad. Despite its lack of meat, it consisted of highly spiced foods such as curries. In addition, Indians used stimulants including tobacco, liquor, and opium. Moreover, and even more telling, the Indians were notorious for being "exceedingly indolent, sensual, and licentious." In India, Graham reported, "we see excesses of every kind committed without hesitation, and boys of very tender age freely allowed to ramble over nights and nights, and spend hours and hours in immoral pursuits." To satisfy their "effeminate lust," it was not uncommon for young Indian men to go, oftentimes intoxicated, "upon the river with their lewd companions, and revel in all sorts of licentiousness." Enmeshed as Graham felt they were in drunkenness, fornication, and even homosexuality, he was not surprised that these people were the first to be ravaged by cholera.[32]

Diet and sex, then, were the areas that most frequently debilitated the system of organic life. It was plain, Graham claimed, that "in the whole career of the epidemic cholera, dietetic intemperance and lewdness have been the grand purveyors to its devastating rage. In every country, the drunken and the lewd have fallen almost by hundreds and by thousands before this terrible destroyer!" Consider the fact that "out of fourteen hundred lewd women [i.e., prostitutes] in one street in Paris, thirteen hundred died of cholera" when the epidemic hit that city. Indeed, "in a single house, sixty of these wretched creatures perished by this disease."[33] There are people, Graham noted, who mistakenly attribute such phenomena to the fact that most prostitutes are forced, because of their poverty, to subsist on a "meagre diet" which weakens and debilitates their bodies, and renders them susceptible to disease. But Graham insisted that this explanation was inadequate: while it is true that prostitutes are invariably debilitated, their state does not stem from the meagerness of their diet. "In the first place, ninety-nine hundredths of those unfortunate creatures, are excessive in their use of intoxicating substances." But it is not their drinking habits alone that render prostitutes particularly susceptible to cholera; it is the very nature of their chosen profession.

> The debility induced by excessive lewdness, is always far more the result of excessive excitement and irritation than of any other cause; and the alimentary canal is almost invariably the very first to suffer from these irritations, and to be brought into a state of debility, morbid irritability, and even inflammation; and not infrequently, the very worst of gastritis and enteritis are induced by excesses of this kind.[34]

Like alcohol, spices, and animal food, then, the "excitement" of sexual activity was able to provoke irritation, inflammation, and organic debility. Sexual feelings, like the desire for food and drink—like all the "natural appetites," in other words—were harmless and even healthy as long as "exercise and indulgence are kept strictly within the range of their constitutional design." But, when people disregard the "constitutional laws" on which these appetites are established—when they "yield to an excess of their indulgence"—then these same appetites "inevitably become the agents of disease and suffering to us"; and they become so precisely to "the extent to which their indulgence has transgressed the constitutional laws of propriety."[35]

Graham made it wholly clear, even in this 1832 lecture, that it was not only prostitutes whose activities transgressed the constitutional laws of propriety—indeed, that these laws proscribed more than promiscuity alone. "It is not only the openly intemperate and the illicit, that injure themselves by their improper indulgences." Marriage itself does not protect a person from these dangers. In a state of sexual excitement, the human body cannot distinguish a spouse from a lover, or even from client:

> No forms of civil law, or institutions of society, can save us from the evils which result from transgressing the constitutional laws of our nature. All excesses, therefore, beyond the real wants of our system, and the purposes of our organization—and equally when committed within or without the pale of civil institutions—are dangerous to our bodily health and existence.[36]

NOTES

1. *Genius of Temperance*, April 6, 1831; June 1 and 15, 1831; Aug. 31, 1831; Nov. 16, 1831; Sylvester Graham, *Lectures on the Science of Human Life*, 2 vols. (Boston, 1839), 1: vi. See also Edith Cole, "Sylvester Graham, Lecturer on the Science of Human Life: The Rhetoric of a Dietary Reformer" (Ph.D. diss., Indiana University), pp. 65-69. Graham also lectured at the Hicksite Quaker meetinghouse in Salem, N.J., and in the nearby town of Bridgeton.

2. John Bell and D. Francis Condie, *All the material facts in the history of epidemic cholera: being a report of the College of Physicians of Philadelphia, to the Board of Health: and a full account of the causes, post mortem appearances, and treatment of the disease* (Philadelphia, 1832). Condie and Bell were also co-editors of the *Journal of Health*. A second edition of the report appeared later the same year. For an account and analysis of the contemporary literature about

cholera, and a history of the epidemic itself, see Charles Rosenberg, *The Cholera Years* (Chicago, 1962), pp. 1-98; and Charles Rosenberg, "The Cause of Cholera: aspects of etiological thought in nineteenth century America," *Bulletin of the History of Medicine*, 34 (1960): 331-354, esp. pp. 331-338.

3. *Genius of Temperance*, June 27, 1832; Cole, "Sylvester Graham," p. 71.

4. Bell and Condie, *Epidemic Cholera*, pp. 93-94, 127, 130-31. Bell and Condie also recommended leeches. Sylvester Graham, *A Lecture on Epidemic Diseases Generally, and Particularly the Spasmodic Cholera, delivered in . . . New York, March, 1832* (New York, 1833). I have used the second (Boston, 1838) edition of this work, in which Graham's condemnation of drugs can be found on pp. 38-42.

5. By mid-1832 Graham's followers were being called "Grahamites"—a sure sign of popular success. Graham collected many of his followers' testimonials (which generally were recorded in terms similar to those characteristic of religious conversions during the same period) and published them as *The Aesculapian Tablets of the Nineteenth Century* (Providence, 1834). It was at this time, too, that he brought out his edition of Luigi Cornaro's *Discourses on a Sober and Temperate Life* (New York, 1833)—itself the record of a "conversion."

Two recent studies which discuss American medicine in the antebellum years deal with Graham only briefly. Joseph Kett and William Rothstein are mainly interested in how Graham's ideas about preventive medicine and hygiene supplemented the critique of conventional "heroic" medical practice developed by medical sects such as the Thomsonians. See William Rothstein, *American Physicians in the Nineteenth Century* (Baltimore, 1972), pp. 158-159, and Joseph F. Kett, *The Formation of the American Medical Profession, 1780-1860* (New Haven, 1968), pp. 122-126.

6. F. J. V. Broussais, *Cholera, Two Clinical Lectures upon the Nature, Treatment, and Symptoms of Spasmodic Cholera. Delivered during the Prevalence of the Disease in Paris* (New York, 1832).

7. Graham, *Cholera*, pp. iii, iv.

8. Ibid., p. 5. Bichat had written that "life is the totality of those functions which resist death."

9. Ibid., p. 5.

10. The quotations in this paragraph and the two preceding paragraphs can be found in ibid., pp. 7-9.

11. For a more extensive examination of the differences between Bichat's and Graham's treatment of the relationship between animal and organic life, see chapter 8.

12. Graham, *Cholera*, pp. 6, 9-10. The primacy of the organic system was apparent, Graham suggested (employing an observation Bichat had made before him, although for another purpose), from the fact that while organic life can function normally when animal life has been interrupted or disturbed—during sleep, for example, or following a stroke—the converse does not hold: "animal life cannot continue an instant after organic life is destroyed." For that reason organic life is more crucial than animal (p. 10).

13. Ibid., p. 11. While Graham acknowledged that the stomach is not "the source of nervous energy to the system," he nevertheless insisted that its "nervous supply" was so rich that "it may with propriety be considered the common index of the whole system." See also p. 21.

14. Ibid., pp. 12-13, 21.

15. Ibid., pp. 12-13, 16.

16. Ibid., pp. 12-13.

17. Ibid.

18. Ibid., pp. 14-16.

19. Ibid., pp. 16-17.

20. Ibid., pp. 18, 23-24.

21. Ibid., pp. 18, 22-24, 38.

22. Ibid., p. 23. "Atmospheric changes" and "noxious gases or effluvia" were the commonest explanations of the etiology of cholera at the time of the 1832 epidemic. See Rosenberg, *Cholera Years*, p. 75; and Rosenberg, "The Cause of Cholera," pp. 331-338. What Graham was suggesting, in other words, was that while atmospheric changes, etc., might indeed be responsible for the disease, their role was merely that of catalyst. It was characteristic of Graham's intellectual imprecision that he interpreted the use of artificial stimulants both as the habit which predisposed the body to disease and as the catalyst which set it off. "The primary cause," he says at another point, "is always the peculiar condition of the human system, resulting from the violation of the laws of organic life. Its more immediately exciting causes, however, are various; such as atmospheric changes and conditions—quality and quantity of food—excesses of every kind; but more than all, perhaps, the excesses of filthy sensuality, and the use of artificial stimulants" (p. 26).

23. Graham, *Cholera*, pp. 27-36. These were the years of religious revivals led by Charles G. Finney.

24. Ibid., pp. 44-46. In arguing that cholera was not contagious, Graham was once again in substantial agreement with the majority of American medical men of his day. According to Rosenberg, out of a randomly selected group of 109 American physicians whose views on the subject can be determined, 90 denied that cholera was at all contagious. This fits in, of course, with the prevalent opinion that the epidemic was the product of atmospheric changes. (Roughly one-half of those 90 physicians blamed the epidemic on such changes.) Rosenberg, *Cholera Years*, p. 75.

25. Gerald F. Pyle, "The Diffusion of Cholera in the United States in the Nineteenth Century," *Geographical Analysis*, 1 (1969): 59-75. See also Allan R. Pred, *Urban Growth and the Circulation of Information: The United States System of Cities 1790-1840* (Cambridge, 1973), pp. 245-246. Pred demonstrates an intriguing correlation between the diffusion of the cholera epidemic and the spread of the suspension of specie payments by American banks five years later during the Panic of 1837 (pp. 246-255).

26. "It is worthy of remark," Graham wrote, "that this dreadful epidemic appears to be peculiarly a disease of the organic domain. Animal life is seldom very much affected by it . . . and the brain, in particular, is seldom so much distracted as to disorder the mental manifestations." *Cholera*, p. 25.

27. Ibid., pp. 48-50.

28. Ibid., pp. 58-59, 70-72; see also p. 74.

29. Ibid., pp. 54, 57-58.

30. Ibid., pp. 55-56, 58.

31. Ibid., pp. 58-59. For persons already ill with cholera Graham recommended an even stricter and more reduced version of the same diet. (Meat, for instance, is forcefully and unequivocally forbidden to such persons.) For Graham's therapeutic recommendations, see Graham, *Cholera*, pp. 38-44.

32. Ibid., pp. 60-62.

33. Ibid., p. 49; see also p. 69. Graham picked up these bits of information, like many of the other "facts" that appear in the course of the *Lecture*, from newspapers. See Rosenberg, *Cholera Years*, p. 41. Rosenberg suggests that many people made the connection between cholera and sexual excess at this time (pp. 41-42). Paris, which, in fact was hard hit by the epidemic, was in Graham's eyes a quagmire of moral filth. On several occasions he contrasted it unfavorably with London. In addition to his comparison of the drinking habits of the citizens of the two cities, Graham noted that English food was "far more simple and natural" than French, and that "for excessive lewdness, which is another powerful, predisposing cause of cholera, Paris has long been exceedingly notorious." In corroboration of this judgment he cited statistics dealing with illegitimate births in that city. Graham, *Cholera*, pp. 68-69.

34. Graham, *Cholera*, p. 50; see also pp. 35-36.

35. Ibid., p. 49.

36. Ibid., p. 51.

7. SEX: THE PATHOLOGY OF DESIRE

In his lecture on cholera, Sylvester Graham made it clear that there was a close connection between sexual excess and disease, but in that essay he merely hinted at the nature of the connection and did not try to describe it in any detail. Only in *Lecture to Young Men on Chastity,* published in 1834 (but first delivered as early as April 1832 to the largest audience he had addressed until that time),[1] did Graham systematically address himself to the question. On this occasion he chose to spend little time in expounding the principles of Bichat and Broussais. Nevertheless, those principles pervaded Graham's analysis of human sexuality in its normal and its diseased manifestations.

Sexuality, as Graham explained it, is associated with both organic and animal life. The ability of the male generative organs, for instance, to produce semen and to "eject it with peculiar convulsions," is a function of organic life while the voluntary physical movement of the penis during sexual acts is a function of animal life. Because of its dual nature, the reproductive apparatus alone among the organs of the body is integrally connected both to the brain and to the digestive system—and, indeed, it forms a direct link between the two.

The brain and the genital organs exert a reciprocal influence on each other. On the one hand, "lascivious thoughts and imaginations" can easily "excite and stimulate" the genital system by increasing the flow of blood in their direction and thus increasing their "secretions and peculiar sensibilities." On the other hand, "an excited state of the genital organs"—the product either of diseased action or an abundance of semen in the testes—"will throw its influence upon the brain, and force lascivious thoughts and imaginations upon the mind."

A similar "reciprocity of influence" exists between the organs of reproduction and those of digestion. The condition of the stomach, heart, lungs, and skin in large measure determines that of the sexual apparatus; their own state, in turn, is "immediately and strongly affected by the condition of the sexual organs."[2] In this way diseases of both animal and organic life can be transmitted sympathetically to the sexual organ. Irritations of the brain, Graham believed, commonly result in a "diseased prurience": individuals suffering from "nervous melancholy" are often "morbidly lecherous," and insanity itself is "generally attended with excessive sexual desire." (It is for this reason, Graham noted, that "many people, who were perfectly modest when in health, become exceedingly obscene, in their conduct and talk, when insane; and often, if they are not prevented, give themselves up to self-pollution.") In the same way, irritations of the alimentary canal, generally induced by improper diet, result in increased sexual desire. "All kinds of stimulating and heating substances, high-seasoned food, rich dishes, the free use of flesh, and even the excess of aliment . . . increase the concupiscent excitability and sensibility of the genital organs."[3]

Just as lust is brought on by disease, so disease is brought on by lust. Sexual desire affects every organ in the body, and "when it kindles into a passion, its influence is so extensive and powerful, that it disturbs and disorders all the functions of the system." It obstructs digestion and respiration, while simultaneously accelerating circulation so that "an increased quantity of blood is injected into the brain, stomach, lungs, and other important organs." In due course there results a "general debility and increased irritability of the nerves of organic life." The vital energy of the system is diminished, and both physical and mental powers are seriously impaired.[4]

At the same time, diseased prurience often leads to increased sexual activity. When this is the case, according to Graham, its effects may include:

> languor, lassitude, muscular relaxation, general debility and heaviness, depression of spirits, loss of appetite, indigestion, faintness and sinking at the pit of the stomach, increased susceptibilities of the skin and lungs to all the atmospheric changes, feebleness of circulation, chilliness, headache, melancholy, hypochondria, hysterics, feebleness of all the senses, impaired vision, loss of sight,

weakness of the lungs, nervous cough, pulmonary consumption, disorders of the liver and kidneys, urinary difficulties, disorders of the genital organs, spinal diseases, weakness of the brain, loss of memory, epilepsy, insanity, apoplexy;—abortions, premature births, and extreme feebleness, morbid predispositions, and early death of offspring. . . .[5]

Over the course of thirty pages Graham graphically traced the effects of venereal excess on the human body and mind, organ by organ. Most severely affected, of course, was the stomach. Digestion was the first physiological process to suffer the effects of sexual excess: the appetite becomes "capricious"; there is constant pain, often "dull and gnawing" but occasionally "acute and shooting"; and an "indescribable sensation of sinking, death-like faintness, attended frequently with a distressing fluttering, or spasmodic affections, will be experienced in the same region, almost without intermission." Finally a "general sense of languor, and debility, and exhaustion" will occur—a feeling which resembles "confirmed dyspepsia"—and in some cases "acute inflammation, and morbid sensibility, of the most excruciating and dangerous character, will suddenly take place."[6]

Similarly, the heart and circulatory system participate in the "diffused excitement of the sexual organs" and suffer thereby from their own "convulsive efforts, and distensions, and repeated irritations." Because of this disruption, the circulation becomes "very feeble and languid," and the results are "emaciation, lassitude, general chilliness, coldness of the extremities, and great debility." When persons in such a condition are so imprudent as to engage in sexual activity, they may have heart attacks: "the violent convulsive paroxysms attending the acme of venereal indulgence, often cause spasms in the heart . . . sometimes producing aneurisms, or bursting of its walls, and suffering the blood to gush out into the pericardium; and causing sudden death, in the unclean act."

The lungs, too, "suffer the common excitement and debility of the whole nervous system, from the acts of venereal indulgence." Their irritation often results in asthma, hoarseness, and "dry, hacking cough." Worst of all, Graham claimed, is pulmonary consumption, or tuberculosis, which is aggravated where it already exists and induced where it does not, by venereal excess of all types—"especially in the form of self-pollution." On occasion, when the "over-excited and convulsed heart" pumps blood into the debilitated lungs more rapidly than they can dispose of it, there may follow a "rupture of the vessels, hemmorhage of the lungs, and gushing of blood from the mouth and nostrils." Even tuberculosis could be a sexual ailment!

Other organs are affected by sexual excess in less dramatic but equally dangerous ways. The liver becomes susceptible to jaundice, and the kidneys to diabetes. In some cases the presence of urine "tortures the morbidly sensitive neck of the bladder" and produces "spasmodic affections and stranguary"; ulcerations commonly take place as well, accompanied by "purulent discharges from the penis." The muscles become weakened, the bones "dry and brittle," the teeth loose and decayed, the bodily fluids "crude, acrid and irritating." The skin ceases to perspire freely: it accumulates impurities instead of expelling them, and it soon becomes a repository of boils, blisters, and pimples "of a livid hue." At the same time it "loses its healthy, clear and fresh appearance, and assumes a sickly, pale, shrivelled, turbid and cadaverous aspect"—invariably a telling mark of the sexual offender. (Here was the origin of the belief that teenage acne was evidence of masturbation.)

In this entire process, Graham continued, the "grand medium of injury" to the rest of the system, and among the worst sufferers itself, is the nervous system. The nerves, especially those of organic life, are simultaneously debilitated and "tortured into a diseased irritability and sensibility." Their vital properties are impaired, along with their "special nervous properties"—the five senses. The sense of touch becomes "obtuse and less discriminating," often to the point of general numbness. The sense of taste is blunted and loses "that delicate perception of agreeable qualities on which the delightful relish of proper and healthful food depends." (It was this problem that was responsible for the widespread "unnatural demand for vicious culinary preparations and stimulating condiments.") The sense of smell is similarly impaired: the olefactory organ "loses its nice discriminating power, and but faintly perceives the rich fragrance which the vegetable kingdom breathes forth for man's enjoyment." The ear grows "dull and hard of hearing." Finally, the eyes become "languid and dull, and lose their brightness and loveliness of expression," and eventually take on a "glassy and vacant appearance." Sight "becomes feeble, obscure, cloudy, confused, and often is entirely lost."

Even the brain is far from immune to the consequences of venereal excess. First, it actually "participates" in sexual excitement in its role as "a mere animal organ," and for this reason both epilepsy and apoplexy are commonly the fate of masturbators and libertines. The brain is equally sensitive, moreover, in its role as the center of the mental and moral faculties. Sexual excesses, therefore, cause the mind to become "exceedingly carnal," and by degrees it loses the ability to concentrate on ordinary day-to-day responsibilities. "All systematic discipline and education becomes extremely irksome to it." Its "powers of application, and perception, and reflection, continually diminish, and memory slowly decays." For a man in such condition, sex itself has become the only object of attention: "his imagination is constantly filled with lewd and obscene images," and his "morbid lust" recurs in the midst of even the most mundane activities. Almost every object he looks at takes on sexual associations; indeed, "his eye can scarcely fall, by accident, on the sexual parts of any female animal, without awakening a train of obscene thoughts, and exciting a foul concupiscence." The ultimate result is either "habitual depression" or a state of total idiocy.[7]

Such, then, was the extent of the potentially lethal reciprocity between sexual excess and disease—a reciprocity derived from the structure of the nervous system and its role in the transmission of vital energy throughout the body. But this relationship, as Graham describes it, was implicitly more than one of reciprocity: it was also one of metaphoric and real identity. Venery, in Graham's vision, does not merely *produce* disease; it *is* itself a form of disease. It is as unnatural in its origins as any other illness, induced by identical causes and practices (dietary irregularity, for instance), and symptomatically analogous to a bevy of pathological phenomena.

Although this equivalence was not something Graham asserted directly, it is striking that he described pathological processes in quasisexual terms. He spoke of the unhealthy heart, for instance, as being "irritated and distended" by sexual excess, and subject during the "convulsive paroxysms" of the orgasm to "convulsive efforts and spasms" of its own—spasms that result in the "bursting of its walls" and the sudden "gushing out" of the blood, and finally in death. The sexual orgasm, in other words, is paralleled by another (and more immediately lethal) orgasm of the heart: a heart attack.

Graham employs similar language to describe the pathology of the lungs, which, as he says, "suffer the common excitement" produced by sexual indulgence: they, too, are liable to rupture and hemmorhage, ending in the "gushing of blood from the mouth and nostrils." Venereal indulgence can also affect the brain by producing apoplexy (a rupturing of the cerebral vessels) or epilepsy (spasmodic convulsions of the entire body). Like blood, other bodily fluids, including even urine, can take on the role of semen in Graham's pathological allegories of detumescence.

But of all the organs, it is naturally the stomach whose pathological manifestations resemble most closely the venereal activity that so frequently brings them on. In his *Lecture on Cholera,* Graham described the symptoms of that disease—the "spasmodic" cholera, as it was commonly known—in an extended sequence of not altogether consistent but supremely suggestive images. Whenever harmful dietary or sexual practices, he wrote, have created a condition of "excessive morbid irritability" in the organic nervous system, then the gastrointestinal irritation (ordinarily minor in itself) that brings on an attack of cholera becomes suddenly "overwhelming" in intensity, and the entire alimentary canal becomes "an abnormal centre of action to the whole domain of organic nerves." Nervous energy is "distracted" from other parts of the system, and all the other organs are correspondingly "paralyzed." Under these circumstances breathing becomes labored and difficult, and the skin is covered with moisture. "The blood thickens, grows dark and sizy." At the same time, "all that can flow in the system, rushes, in horrid anarchy, to the centre," and produces "the most violent congestion in the vessels leading to the alimentary canal." This congestion, in turn, produces "an intense heat and excitability of the parts, and inundat[es] the stomach and intestines with a most excruciating serous fluid, which tortures beyond measure, the highly irritated and now keenly sensitive mucous membrane which lines them." There follows a period of "violent vomiting and purging," during which "all the muscles of voluntary and involuntary motion [are] thrown into the most violent and painful spasms and convulsions." Total exhaustion ensues, and, if the spasms have been too violent for the system to bear, death.[8]

The orgastic language Graham employed to describe an attack of cholera becomes especially striking when juxtaposed with the curiously similar terms in which he pictured the sexual orgasm itself:

> The convulsive paroxysms attending venereal indulgence, are connected with the most intense excitement, and cause the most powerful agitation to the whole system that it is ever subject to. The brain, stomach, heart, lungs, liver, skin, and the other organs,

feel it sweeping over them with the tremendous violence of a tornado. The powerfully excited and convulsed heart drives the blood, in fearful congestion, to the principal viscera,—producing oppression, irritation, debility, rupture, inflammation, and sometimes disorganization;—and this violent paroxysm is generally succeeded by great exhaustion, relaxation, lassitude and even protraction.[9]

To make these associations is not to engage in a pseudo-Freudian symbol hunt. The point is not that Graham (much like the habitual masturbator he himself described) found sexual connotations everywhere he looked. More significant is the converse point—that he associated sex itself with pain and disease. Lust and orgasm elicited in him images of excruciating membranes, bursting blood vessels, spasmodic seizures, and, especially, digestive discomfort, vomiting and diarrhoea.

This connection helps explain the fact that Graham structured his career after 1831 around the dual problems of digestive and sexual health. What mattered was not merely that the gastrointestinal system and the genital system mutually *affected* each other, even though they surely did, but also that when either of these two systems became irritated and diseased, both responded in similar ways. For Sylvester Graham, "dyspepsia" and venery were simply two modes of diseased action in the organic system of life.

Both orgasm and diarrhoea resulted in the violent discharge of bodily matter through a series of "convulsive spasms." But while Graham may have found this phenomenon disturbing, he also stressed that it was not the cause of the most serious damage wrought by digestive or sexual disturbances. The loss of semen, in particular, was of relatively minor consequence. On this point Graham took pains to dispute the position of such earlier authors as Samuel Tissot, who had claimed[10] that the loss of this fluid was the single most dangerous aspect of sexual abuse. Paraphrasing Tissot without citing him by name, Graham wrote:

> We are told by some writers on this important subject that the genital secretion, or the semen, may be called the essential oil of animal liquors—the rectified spirit—the most subtile and spirituous part of the animal frame, which contributes to the support of the nerves; that the greatest part of this refined fluid is, in a healthy state and conduct of the system, re-absorbed and mixed with the blood, of

which it constitutes the most rarified and volatile part, and imparts to the body peculiar sprightliness, vivacity, muscular strength, and general vigor and energy to the animal machine; that it causes the beard, hair and nails to grow,—gives depth of tone, and masculine scope and power to the voice,—and manliness and dignity to the countenance and person; and energy, and ardor, and noble daring to the mind; and that therefore the emission of semen enfeebles the body more than the loss of twenty times the same quantity of blood,—more than violent cathartics and emetics:—and hence the frequent and excessive loss of it cannot fail to produce the most extreme debility, and disorder, and wretchedness, of both body and mind.'[11]

While Graham acknowledged that semen, "like all other secretions," was to some extent re-absorbed by the body, he insisted that "the importance of semen to the system, and the evils resulting from the mere loss of it, have been exceedingly overrated, by all who have treated of this subject." In fact, he indicated (in a statement that flatly and shockingly contradicted the claims of any sexual authority then available to him), "all the evils resulting from the abuse of the genital organs, occur, in their worst and most incorrigible forms, *where there is no secretion and emission of semen.*"[12]

Orgasm is not required, in other words, to sustain the worst consequences of sexual abuse. The "convulsive paroxysms" that accompany it are, to be sure, substantially more dangerous than the mere emission of semen, but only because they result from "the general tension of the muscles and nervous tissues"—a tension which exists independently of the orgasm that may or may not finally release it. Damage may be done, likewise, by "the flow of blood to the brain, lungs, stomach, and other important organs," but this damage, too, is not contingent on the attainment of climax. In any case, the "grand principle of mischief" lies neither in the muscular paroxysms nor in the movement of the blood, but rather in "*the peculiar excitement of the nervous system*" which inevitably accompanies sexual arousal.[13]

When an individual is sexually excited, Graham wrote, "something very analagous to electricity or galvanism, diffuses a peculiar and powerful excitement throughout the whole nervous system." The exact nature and source of this excitement are as yet uncertain, he acknowledged; it might be produced by a "nervous fluid or spirit," or perhaps by something "still more subtle and intangible." But in any event, it was beyond doubt that this excitement

> is more diffusive, universal, and powerful, than any other to which the system is ever subject; and that it more rapidly exhausts the vital properties of the tissues, and impairs the functional powers of the organs; and consequently that it, in a greater degree than any other cause, deteriorates all the vital processes of nutrition, from beginning to end.[14]

It is "this peculiar EXCITEMENT, or VITAL STIMULATION," and not the orgasm, which "causes the muscular tension and convulsion, and increased action of the heart," and which "occasions visceral congestion, and disturbs all the functions of the system, and thus produces general debility, morbid irritability and sympathy, and all the consequent train of evils which result." It is this excitement which causes blood to rush to the genital organs, and which induces "an increase of their secretions, and of their peculiar sensibilities, sufficient to cause a distraction of functional energy from the digestive, and other organs" (exactly as the external irritation that brings on cholera causes a distraction of functional energy toward the digestive organs); and therefore it is this excitement which manages to "disturb and impair all the functions, and debilitate *all* the organs of the system."

All of these ills can and do come about, Graham reiterated, "without amounting to the acme of coition, and causing an emission of semen, and the convulsive paroxysms which attend it."[15] For this reason, he went on, "SEXUAL DESIRE" alone, "cherished by the mind and dwelt on by the imagination," always and inevitably "throws an influence . . . over the whole nervous domain"—an influence that ultimately produces "irritability, and debility, and relaxation" in the nervous system. "And hence those LASCIVIOUS DAY-DREAMS, and amorous reveries" in which so many persons all-too-frequently indulge, can themselves lead to debility, disease and death, "without the actual exercise of the genital organs!"[16]

It was not only sexual *activity,* then, that suggested disease to Graham: it was also sexual desire itself. As we have seen, Graham frequently referred to desire as something painful—a form of "aching sensibility"— and he insisted that healthy individuals were able to go "for several months in succession" without feeling sexually aroused. Graham based his claim both on empirical examples and on physiological theory. For examples he pointed to the lower animals and to primitive human societies. Most animals, as he reminded his audience, displayed sexual feelings only at widely-spaced intervals, and even then only for short periods of time. For his human example, Graham pointed to those primitive cultures whose members habitually go about entirely naked without ever manifesting any "licentious feelings." It was no coincidence, Graham added, that such primitive peoples generally subsisted on a healthy and stimulant-free vegetable diet.[17]

The scientific principles that explained these examples were to be found in the physiological theory of Xavier Bichat (even though Bichat himself had never applied them to the question of sexual health). Following Bichat, Graham argued that the nerves of organic life were, "in their natural state, entirely destitute of animal sensibility"—and, indeed, that the health and integrity of the organic functions "require such a state of these nerves."[18] But unlike Bichat, Graham considered the nerves that transmitted and registered sexual excitement to be associated exclusively with the organic system of life. For this reason, then, it was possible for him to claim that a healthy organic system implied the general absence of sexual sensations.

In his *Lectures on the Science of Human Life*, published in 1839, Graham made much of the point that people in good health ought never to be aware of any of their bodily operations. "When . . . we are *conscious* that we have a stomach, or a liver from any *feeling* in those organs," he wrote, "we may be certain that something is wrong." In a state of health "there is no *local feeling*—no animal perception of a distinct sensation *in any particular part;* nay indeed, there is not the least animal consciousness of any internal organ."[19] While Graham did not suggest in this passage that he was including sexual desire, along with an aching stomach, as one of the local feelings which indicated that "something is wrong," in the wider context of his intellectual career it is a plausible association to make.

Another indication that Graham considered sexual feelings to be quasi-pathological is the curious way he used the term "debilitation." When an eighteenth-century writer like Samuel Tissot argued that debilitation ("epuisement") was an inevitable consequence of self-abuse, he meant that the practice caused one's bodily strength—sexual and otherwise—to be drained away. In Tissot's view, a man who had masturbated himself into a state of debility would be unable either to function or to feel: he would lose his ability to digest food, for instance, or to perform the sexual act;

and at the same time he would also lose the ability to feel hunger or sexual desire.

In other words, for Tissot, debilitation meant the loss of sensation as well as the loss of potency, and health meant the restoration of both. But for Graham the term had just the opposite implication: along with the loss of power, debilitation meant the *aggravation* of internal feeling, and health meant its disappearance. Graham consistently linked exhaustion with excitement and weakness with irritability, as if the two were merely different modes of a single condition. Thus he could write that after continued sexual excesses, the nervous system is "tortured into a shocking state of debility, and excessive irritability . . . and aching sensibility." (Sensibility was always "aching" to Graham.)

Graham and Tissot agreed that venereal excesses led to impotence and sterility; but while Tissot associated these conditions with the loss of sexual sensation, Graham insisted that they involved the development in the genital organs of "an unhealthy degree of their peculiar sensibility." These organs became, he insisted—and it was a warning he was trying to sound, not a promise—"far more susceptible of excitement" than they would in a state of health. The intensification of desire, in other words, was a punishment for its indulgence. Desire itself was a form of irritation, and irritation was a symptom of debility and disease.[20]

So all-encompassing was Graham's critique of human sexuality that it did not seem to allow for any distinctions at all, quantitative or qualitative. On the basis of his own assumptions, why should masturbation, sodomy, fornication, or adultery be more serious violations of physiological law than ordinary sexual intercourse performed by husband and wife? Taken to their logical conclusion, Graham's arguments came perilously close to condemning marriage itself, and suggesting the physical and moral desirability of total celibacy.[21] Graham himself was able to sense this danger, at least unconsciously, and on one occasion, he moved to head it off.

Earlier books on the subject were of no use to him. The early eighteenth-century author of *Onania,* of course, had never encountered the problem. For him marriage was the one lawful "refuge" from masturbation and similar forbidden practices—a refuge within whose walls no act was wholly forbidden. Tissot, writing later in the eighteenth century, might have been faced with Graham's problem, since both men restricted their arguments to the area of physiology. But Tissot, unlike Graham,

was concerned only with condemning masturbation and not with justifying marriage, and so the problem he faced was not quite the same. Tissot
did not distinguish legitimate from illegitimate forms of sexual intercourse;
instead, he isolated the effects of masturbation from those of *all* forms
of coitus, whether legal or illegal. Tissot made no effort to judge the relative virtues of marital and nonmarital sex—a distinction which even the
author of *Onania* was careful to make. Nor did Tissot argue, as *Onania*
did, that masturbation violated the commands of scripture. (Indeed, he
contemptuously dismissed *Onania* as a "veritable chaos" of "theological
and moral trivialities.") Instead, Tissot condemned masturbation, as
Graham did, solely on the grounds that it had dangerous physical effects,
which he explained by reference to the laws of an abstract and undefined
entity he termed "nature." In moderation, Tissot suggested, nature demands sexual activity. There is a limit to the amount of semen that the
body can hold; and when the testes are full, it is necessary for some of it
to be released. But it is the "destination" of the semen, he insisted, which
"determines the single legitimate means of its evacuation." If the "dangerous consequences" of the loss of semen depended "only on its quantity," Tissot argued, then it would not matter whether ejaculation resulted
from intercourse or from masturbation. But in fact "the form is the root
of this matter." It is true that "very burdensome ills" may also result when
too much semen is lost in natural ways ("les voies de la nature"), but
these ills are far more serious "when the same quantity has been dissipated
in ways that are against nature."[22]

In another place Tissot explained the specific physiological mechanisms
that render masturbation such a uniquely pernicious practice. For one
thing, he noted, masturbation is more commonly provoked by sheer habit
than by physiological need (i.e., the presence of an abundance of semen
in the testes). It is a habit which is particularly easy to develop, since there
are rarely any serious obstacles to its performance. As a solitary habit,
moreover, masturbation has the unfortunate tendency of leading its
practitioners to shun society rather than to seek it.

All these arguments were similar, in fact, to those Graham would employ seventy years later. More unique were Tissot's two parting shots. He
based the first of these on the curious theory, a conventional one in his
day, that all living organisms "transpire" ("transpirent") through count-
less tiny pores in their skin. These pores, he noted, serve both to release
"an extremely fine humor" and to take in "a portion of the fluids which

surround them." In a state of sexual excitement, Tissot argued, all the operations of the body become more intense, and for this reason persons in such a state release, through "transpiration," a greater quantity of this humor than usual—enough of it, in fact, to weaken the body almost as much as the loss of semen itself. But when this increased transpiration takes place in the course of coitus, Tissot went on, the humor is not actually lost; instead, it is exchanged between the two partners. "The one takes in what the other releases." In the course of an onanistic act, however, "the masturbator loses, and recovers nothing." For this reason masturbation is debilitating while coitus is not. Through sexual intercourse, in fact, a strong and healthy individual can help to "reinvigorate" a weaker one, whose own humors stand in need of replenishment. Thus "the young girl who slept with [King] David increased his power." Young girls, conversely, are only weakened by sleeping with old men.[23]

The final difference "between those who are drawn to women, and masturbators," in Tissot's view, lay in the contrast between "the joy which grips the soul" during coitus and the "purely corporeal lust" that characterizes masturbation. While Tissot acknowledged that there is nothing intrinsically harmful about this corporeal lust, he argued that the spiritual joy accompanying intercourse actually provides a variety of gratuitous physiological benefits: it "aids digestion, enlivens circulation, improves all the functions, and replenishes and sustains the powers of the body." Tissot cited one writer who went so far as to claim that it was healthier for a man to make love to an attractive woman than to an ugly one. "And is it possible to doubt," Tissot concluded, "that nature would attach greater good to pleasures gained by means which are her own ("dans ses voies") than by those means which are repugnant to her?"[24]

These arguments were simply not available for Graham to use. Since he condemned nonmarital intercourse as well as masturbation, he needed to find a line of reasoning that would distinguish limited marital sex from both of these practices, as Tissot's argument clearly did not. It was a difficult job. In fact, Graham was unable to devise a single approach that made the necessary distinctions in a convincing way—such arguments would emerge only in the 1840s. He chose, therefore, to argue each count separately: to show in one place why masturbation was "the worst form of sexual indulgence," and in another place why illicit coitus was more harmful than intercourse between husband and wife.

On the first of these issues, of course, Graham avoided anything resembling Tissot's final two points. He did argue, much as Tissot had argued before him, that masturbation was particularly dangerous because "it is a secret and solitary vice, which requires the consent of no second person, and therefore . . . has little to prevent its frequency." For this reason, he added, it is "generally commenced very early in life"—often well before puberty. It was in fact the public schools—"and especially boarding-schools and colleges"—that were the worst breeding grounds of the vice.

Graham condemned mastrubation, finally, as "wholly unnatural." This was a notion, of course, that Tissot had used as well. But Graham intended something quite specific by it, and not just an appeal to the general principle of "nature." Masturbation, Graham argued, is a "forced effect" which involves the "concentrated energy of all the powers of the human system." Unlike coitus, it requires the active and strained participation of the imagination before it can be accomplished. It demands the "mental action, and power of imagination [operating] on the genital organs"; and this action establishes "reciprocal influences between the brain and genital organs"—reciprocal influences that are entirely unnatural and debilitating. As a result, the genital organs regularly become excited by the brain and not as a result of their own needs (for instance, an abundance of semen). In this way a vicious cycle is created from which it is impossible to escape.[25]

This last point served as the basis of Graham's insistence that "illicit commerce between the sexes" was "more injurious, in a physical point of view, than the commerce between man and wife." The difference between nonmarital and marital sex, he argued, stems from the very fact that "it is not the mere loss of semen, but the peculiar excitement, and the violence of the convulsive paroxysms, which produces the mischief, and these are exceedingly increased by the actions of the mind." When males are about to engage in illicit sexual ventures, Graham suggested, they "generally contemplate the act for a considerable time before its performance"; and as a consequence "their imagination is wrought up, and presents lewd and exciting images,—the genital organs become stimulated, and throw their peculiar influence over the whole system." What happens, in other words, is similar to what happens in the case of masturbation: a reciprocal action is established between the mind and the genital organs, so that sexual excitement is sustained not by the internal needs of the system but by the operations of a diseased imagination. "The sight, or touch of the female body, and especially the bosom, etc., greatly increase the excitement." The excitement continues to increase in intensity, the more so "in proportion to the difficulties in the way." Under these circumstances, when "indulgence" finally does take place, "the excitement is intense and overwhelming, and the convulsive paroxysms proportionally violent and hazardous to life."

When a man is sexually "promiscuous," the situation becomes even more dangerous. For such a man the genitals are "almost continually stimulated by the mind." Nearly every female becomes an "object of desire," and "the contemplation of her charms, and all her movements, increases the lust." In this way "the genital organs are kept under an habitual excitement," which is in turn "reflected or diffused over the entire nervous system," and which "disturbs and disorders all the functions of the body . . . and leads to that frequency of commerce which produces the most ruinous consequences."

"But, between husband and wife," Graham argued in what must surely pass as one of the more unusual justifications of marriage ever offered, "all these causes either entirely lose, or are exceedingly diminished in their effect." Marital sex, he reported, was simply not as exciting as nonmarital sex. After a time together the married couple "become accustomed to each other's body, and their parts no longer excite an impure imagination." They are not continually stimulated by the thought or the sight of each other. For this reason, when they make love "their sexual intercourse is the result of the more natural and instinctive excitements of the organs themselves." Graham added that when "their dietetic and other habits are such as they should be, this intercourse is very seldom." In this way, he concluded, marriage provides for "the highest welfare of man." Far from constituting an arbitrary arrangement enforced by society, the "permanent and exclusive connection of one man with one woman is . . . founded in the constitutional nature of things."[26]

When he spoke of "correct" dietetic habits, Graham was referring, of course, to vegetable diet; and it was in the *Lecture on Chastity* that Graham first came to advocate, at least in print, a universal vegetarianism. He had, to be sure, warned against the use of animal food two years earlier in his *Lecture on Cholera*, but whatever his private inclinations may have been at the time, he had explicitly stated then that he intended his warning to apply only "during the prevalence of malignant and epidemic diseases." But unlike cholera, prurience did not sweep over the world in the form of an occasional epidemic. It was present, at least in "civilized" societies, at all times, and in order to subdue it, vegetable diet had to become a permanent habit of life. Graham wrote:

> The truth of the matter is simply this—a pure and well regulated vegetable diet, serves to take away or prevent all morbid or preternatural sexual lust, and to bring and keep the instinct more in a truly natural state, and in strict accordance with the final cause of man's sexual organization, and thus enable him to be chaste in body and spirit.[27]

The "other" habits to which Graham alluded were those of personal hygiene. The strength and tone of the body had to be maintained, not by artificial stimulants but by "active exercise." If a man wished both to subdue his lust and to maintain his strength in the face of a radically reduced diet, then "let him go to the gymnasium," Graham argued: "let him swing upon and climb the poles, and ropes, and ladders, and vault upon the wooden horse." Better still, let him simply "walk, and run, and jump, or labor on the farm." If he was able, let him ride on horseback too. ("But if horseback riding causes involuntary emissions," Graham added in a footnote to the text, "this mode of exercise must be avoided.") In short, he argued, it was necessary to avoid "sedentary habits," because these habits cause blood to gather in "the lower parts of the body, including the genital organs."[28] It was equally necessary to avoid all "anxieties and excitements of the mind," for there were "special sympathies and reciprocities" that connected the genital organs to the brain as well as to the alimentary canal; and mental excitement was as disruptive of sexual serenity as animal food. For this reason it was even necessary to avoid "the disproportionate exercise of the brain in the cultivation of the mind." Graham warned of the harm that could be done, especially to young people, by devoting too much time to study and not enough to physical exercise. Overly intense mental effort caused the brain to become "oppressed, over-heated, weakened, and rendered too excitable." Since the brain is intimately connected with the sexual organs, "a preternatural sensibility, excitability and prurience are increased in these organs too."

Graham was opposed, as Rousseau had been opposed seventy years earlier, to forcing formal education on young children. To insure their sexual health as well as their general well-being, he insisted that it was necessary to "abandon our attempts at early education, and turn our children loose, to develope [sic] their bodies like calves and colts." Along with modern manufacturers of the breakfast cereals that are the commercial descendants of his own idealized recipes, Sylvester Graham wanted each of his readers to function like "a healthy animal."[29]

NOTES

1. Sylvester Graham, *A Lecture to Young Men, on Chastity, intended also for the serious consideration of parents and guardians* (Providence, 1834). In his preface to the *Lecture*, dated March 25, 1834, Graham reported that he was prompted to publish it by "the unanimous expression of the opinion, in the American Lyceum in New York, in May last [i.e. 1833], that such a work was wanted, more than any other." In its published form the *Lecture on Chastity* went through ten editions between 1834 and 1848, and it was translated into several languages. For the date at which Graham first lectured on this subject, see *Genius of Temperance*, April 18, 1832.

2. Graham, *Chastity*, pp. 42-44.

3. Ibid., pp. 45-47; see also pp. 79-80, 86. Insane asylums, Graham claimed, were notorious hotbeds of masturbation. Others agreed with him: Samuel B. Woodward, who published a masturbation pamphlet entitled *Hints for the Young* (Boston and Worcester, 1838), was director of the Massachusetts Lunatic Asylum at Worcester, Massachusetts, during the 1830s. Woodward even discussed this problem in the annual *Reports* he prepared for the institution between 1834 and 1838. Woodward also wrote a testimonial about Graham's *Lecture on Chastity* which appeared in the later editions of that work.

4. Graham, *Chastity*, pp. 47-49.

5. Ibid., pp. 78-79. This particular list covers only the difficulties "which are caused by sexual excesses between husband and wife," but it is substantially duplicated in other connections throughout the book.

6. This and the following paragraphs are a summary of material found in ibid., pp. 102-132.

7. Graham also described how excess produced such psychological effects as insomnia, melancholia, and guilt.

8. Sylvester Graham, *A Lecture on Epidemic Diseases Generally, and Particularly the Spasmodic Cholera, delivered in . . . New York, March, 1832* (New York, 1833), pp. 24-25.

9. Graham, *Chastity*, pp. 49-50. In another place Graham speaks of the sexually stimulated body as a "living volcano"—an image somewhat more apt, perhaps, than that of a tornado. It is interesting that Graham, along with other Victorian sexual

theorists, shared with later psychologists and writers such as Wilhelm Reich and D.H. Lawrence a certainty that the sexual orgasm is the most powerful and significant event in human experience.

10. S. A. A. Tissot, *L'Onanisme* (Lausanne, 1760). This book, which had quickly achieved a reputation throughout Europe as the standard treatment of the subject, was not published in America until 1832. It is evident that Graham read it at that time, since he claimed in 1834 that he published his own *Lecture on Chastity* partly in response to the "several works on this subject, in English print . . . every one of [which] is factually erroneous in its physiological views" (*Lecture on Chastity*, pp. 13-14). Since it is to one of Tissot's basic premises that Graham takes particular exception, it presumably was the Swiss physician he had in mind.

11. Graham, *Chastity*, pp. 51-52. Compare the following passage from Tissot:

> The seminal liquor . . . influences so powerfully the forces of the body, and the perfection of digestion which sustains them, that physicians throughout the ages have unanimously believed that the loss of one ounce of this humor is more enfeebling than that of forty ounces of blood. One is able to get an idea of its importance by observing the effects it produces from the time it begins to be formed; the voice, the physiognomy, even the character of the face changes, the beard appears, the whole body often assumes a different air, because the muscles acquire a bulk and strength which produces a sensible difference between the body of an adult and that of a young man who has not reached puberty. . . . Can one doubt, after this, the force of its action on the whole body, and not feel equally how much misfortune the profusion of so precious a humour must bring on? Tissot, *L'Onanisme* (Paris, 1820 ed.), pp. 14-15 (my translation). See also pp. 72-83 ("Importance de la liqueur seminale").

Tissot's essay reflects a curious combination of eighteenth-century mechanism—he constantly speaks of the human body as an "animal machine" which obeys laws similar to those governing the inanimate world—and the classical humoralism that is so apparent in his discussion of the semen as an "essential humor" of the body. Both his mechanism and his humoralism place him in direct contrast with Graham. (In fact, it is the inclusion of the phrase "animal machine" in Graham's garbled quotation that makes it fairly clear that he was attempting to refute Tissot's views.)

12. Graham, *Chastity*, pp. 52, 54 (italics added). Except for Edith Cole's 1975 dissertation, the only serious modern study of Graham's career suggests that he derived his sexual theories directly from Tissot. See William B. Walker, "The Health Reform Movement in the United States, 1830-1870" (Ph.D. diss., Johns Hopkins University, 1955), p. 4. Walker's suggestion was picked up and transformed into an accusation of plagarism by Gerald Carson in his popular study of American vegetarianism and the rise of the breakfast cereal industry, *Cornflake Crusade* (New York, 1957), p. 46. It should be clear that an actual comparison of Graham and Tissot does not confirm this idea.

13. Graham, *Chastity*, pp. 54-55. The italics are Graham's.

14. Ibid., p. 57. Graham's vagueness about the nature of nervous function was not idiosyncratic. Instead it reflected the variety of competing theories that had been advanced during the eighteenth and early nineteenth centuries, theories whose relative merits had not been decided at the time of Graham's own introduction to physiology. For details of representative positions, see Eric T. Carlson and Meribeth M. Simpson, "Models of the Nervous System in 18th Century Psychiatry," *Bulletin of the History of Medicine* 43 (1969): 101-115.

15. Graham, *Chastity*, pp. 57-58. One might conjecture that Graham's unwillingness to admit the importance of semen loss stemmed from his attempt to demonstrate that sexual abuses were as dangerous for women as they were for men. (This was a problem Tissot did not confront since in his day it was believed that women, too, produced a semen-like substance ejaculated during orgasm, and which was necessary to permit conception. See, for instance, Tissot, *L'Onanisme*, pp. 100-101.) But this speculation is inadequate since Graham easily could have claimed that it *was* in fact the "convulsive spasms" of the orgasm that did all the damage. Inasmuch as these spasms were not limited to the male orgasm, he would in this way have accounted adequately enough for women. As I have indicated, of course, Graham employed no such argument. In any case, the *Lecture on Chastity* was intended solely for a male audience as its full title makes clear.

16. Graham, *Chastity*, pp. 58-59.

17. Sylvester Graham, *Lectures on the Science of Human Life*, 2 vols. (Boston, 1839), 2: 646. In his romanticization of non-Western cultures, Graham once again was typical of his generation. Compare, for example, the American Indians in James Fenimore Cooper's later novels, or even many of the blacks in Harriet Beecher Stowe's *Uncle Tom's Cabin*.

18. Graham, *Chastity*, pp. 44, 50, 80.

19. Graham, *Science*, 1: pp. 190, 193.

20. Graham, *Chastity*, pp. 50, 102, 125-126; Tissot, *L'Onanisme*, pp. 136-137, 189-190. This "exponential" function of sexual stimulation was also of great concern to the antimasturbation theorist whom Graham Barker-Benfield has taken as *his* representative Jacksonian reformer, the Reverend John Todd. But while Barker-Benfield is aware of the threat that stimulation in all its forms posed to men such as Todd and Graham, his explanatory model—the "spermatic economy"—does not do complete justice to the physiological importance of the threat.

By focussing too closely on the common belief in a finite pool of bodily energy, available for expenditure in either economic or sexual activity (or any other activity, for that matter), Barker-Benfield is led to overemphasize the degree to which middle-class men tried to achieve economic self-control through the social control of women. For one thing, the pool-of-energy concept evokes a static mercantilist economic universe, and not an expanding capitalist one. For another thing, while Graham and his followers did believe in the pool-of-energy idea, the omnipresent danger that stimulation could provoke a lethal intensification of excitability led Graham to look beyond the social distribution of human energy (i.e., vis-a-vis women) and towards the control of that energy at its very source—the individual mind and body. For his analysis of Todd, see Graham Barker-Benfield, *The Horrors of the Half-Known Life* (New York, 1976), pp. 163-196.

21. It is no coincidence that the celibate Shakers were among the most enthusiastic followers of Graham. See Edward Deming Andrews, *The People called Shakers* (New York, 1953).

22. Tissot, *L'Onanisme*, pp. 15-16, 36-37. Another comment critical of *Onania* can be found on p. 10.

23. Tissot, *L'Onanisme*, pp. 113-115.

24. Ibid., pp. 115-116.

25. Graham, *Chastity*, pp. 87-101. It is significant that these are the only pages in the *Lecture on Chastity* concerned specifically with masturbation. The rest of the work is devoted either to sexual abuse in general or to marital excess in particular.

26. Ibid., pp. 71-75.

27. Ibid., p. 187. While Tissot, like Graham, prescribed a "natural cure" for masturbation, he encouraged the use of animal food for this purpose and he recommended "all meats [taken] from young animals," including veal, lamb, baby beef, chicken, squab, and partridge (*L'Onanisme*, p. 146). As for alcohol, which Graham needless to say proscribed above all other things, Tissot insisted that the best drink for persons trying to get over the masturbation habit was water "mixed with an equal part of wine." The most important rule, Tissot insisted, was to avoid those drinks which tended to "increase feebleness and relaxation"; and if one had to take such drinks, to add a little liquor to them (pp. 159-160). He also advocated the use of certain drugs—Graham condemned them all—such as quinine, which was to be taken, Tissot directed, "with red wine" (p. 184). The contrast that emerges here between Tissot and Graham is a function, of course, of the two men's different assumptions about the physiology of stimulation and debility, which Tissot saw as wholly opposite conditions and which Graham saw as merely different modes of a single condition.

28. In promoting the curative and counteraphrodisiac powers of vigorous exercise Graham was expressing commonplace nineteenth-century hygiene literature. For a representative sampling of similar views see John R. Betts, "American Medical Thought on Exercise as the Road to Health," *Bulletin of the History of Medicine* 45 (1971): 38-58.

29. Graham, *Chastity*, pp. 144-150, 154-155, 162-163.

8. THE SCIENCE OF HUMAN LIFE

After the *Lecture of Chastity* appeared in 1834, Sylvester Graham published nothing more about sex. By 1839, when his two-volume *Lectures on the Science of Human Life* was printed, Graham had come to focus much of his attention on a sensation even more pervasive and often more implacable than sexual desire itself—the sensation of hunger. Graham distrusted hunger much as he distrusted lust, even though he acknowledged that both were indisputably necessary—one for self-preservation and the other for the preservation of the species. Nevertheless, considered purely in themselves, both appetites were volatile and dangerous internal irritations.

Hunger led to what Graham perceived as a kind of erection of the digestive apparatus. When the body is in need of food, he wrote, the stomach, which is normally relaxed and flaccid, is brought into "a particular physiological condition" in which, and only in which, it is capable of fulfilling its natural function. Such a condition involves "a concentration of vital energy" in its own tissues and an "increase of vital stimulus" to the network of nervous tissue that pervades it. As a result, the blood vessels of the stomach "become somewhat more injected with blood, exalting the vital properties of all the other tissues, and preparatory to the secretion of the gastric juice." In addition, the temperature of the organ "is slightly elevated, and the whole organ becomes more red, and has something of an excited appearance." It is in this state of "vital exaltation," Graham concluded—he took the phrase from Broussais—that the stomach "possesses its greatest functional power."[1]

Graham had insisted five years earlier in the *Lecture on Chastity* that lust was "natural" only when the body as a whole was in a healthy condition. Only then, he had argued, did sexual desire reflect "the natural excitements of the organs themselves rather than the unnatural needs of habit or artificial irritation." In just the same way, he now argued that it was only when the body is in "a perfectly normal, healthy and undepraved state" that hunger is "a true, instinctive indication of the alimentary wants of the system." When dietary error has irritated the nerves of organic life and induced in them a "morbid irritability and sympathy," then "the sense of hunger may become a mere demand for accustomed stimulation, and in no degree, indicate the true alimentary wants of the body." In such a case hunger is a "totally blind and exceedingly dangerous guide"— no more reliable a guide to safe eating than "the drunkard's thirst is in regard to drinking." Indeed, Graham warned, "this morbid appetite is always the more despotic and imperious, in proportion as it is removed from the original integrity of the function."[2]

Like other American reformers of his generation, Graham believed, and even insisted, that all natural "instincts" were by definition good and healthful. At the same time he recognized, and maintained even more forcefully, that people generally behaved in a way that was dangerous and destructive. Graham tried, much like his fellow reformers, to resolve this contradiction by insisting that the destructive behavior that pervaded modern society was based not on natural instinct at all, but on a constellation of artificial needs—pseudo-needs—that had been generated by the pressures of modern civilization. Nineteenth-century Americans might crave too much of the wrong kind of food, just as they might crave too much of the wrong kind of sex—but neither of these cravings reflected real physiological needs. True instinct was never "despotic and imperious." (These very words recalled the kind of political perversions from which republican America had liberated itself two generations earlier.) The demands imposed by natural hunger were invariably modest and benign.

Only those people who had already adopted a vegetable diet could know what natural hunger was like: Just as a wife arouses less intense desire and excitement than a mistress, vegetable foods provoke a more moderate kind of hunger than animal foods. The feeling of hunger, Graham argued, is "greater and more imperious in the flesh-eater" than it is in the vegetarian; the appetite of the latter "has nothing of that despotic, vehement and impatient character, which marks the craving desire of the flesh-eater."[3]

Vegetarians have a further advantage over meat-eaters: they are able to skip a meal with equanimity. In fact, they "can even fast for days with comparatively little distress or disquietude."[4] Meat-eaters, in contrast, invariably eat too much, and too often. The voraciousness of meat-eaters was, for Graham, both a symbol and a cause of the problems besetting nineteenth-century society. As he put it, "Excessive alimentation is one of the greatest sources of evil to the human family in civic life."

Graham made the radical reduction of food consumption one of the cardinal principles of his system. It was, in fact, one of the few principles he saw fit to print in capital letters:

> EVERY INDIVIDUAL SHOULD, AS A GENERAL RULE,
> RESTRAIN HIMSELF TO THE SMALLEST QUANTITY,
> WHICH HE FINDS FROM CAREFUL INVESTIGATION AND
> ENLIGHTENED EXPERIENCE AND OBSERVATION, WILL
> FULLY MEET THE ALIMENTARY WANTS OF THE VITAL
> ECONOMY OF HIS SYSTEM,—KNOWING THAT WHATSO-
> EVER IS MORE THAN THIS IS EVIL![5]

Graham's demand for minimal consumption (along with his notorious emphasis on home-baked bread) amounted, quite literally, to a declaration of physical independence from the capitalist marketplace. The unnatural hunger of meat-eaters, like their equally imperious sexual lust, was a symbol as well as a cause of the fact that they—Jacksonian Americans—had lost their self-sufficiency and were coming to be the uncontrolled creatures, the Frankenstein monsters, of what Graham chose to call "civic life."

"Intensive and extensive life are incompatible," Graham commented laconically in a notebook he kept during the 1830s. The more serene a person's existence, the longer it was apt to last—"the more intense the shorter." It was for this very reason, Graham speculated, that people in earlier periods of time lived (as the Bible reported) for so many years. After all, in past times the "vital processes" of the human race were "much less rigid and intense" than they had become subsequently. "Childhood and adolescence" in premodern society were "proportionately protracted, and the change from youth to manhood took place at a much greater remove from birth." But modern life, with its interconnected arsenal of economic, dietary, and emotional stimulants, "accelerates all the functions."[6] Children grow up prematurely, and adults die, exhausted, long before their time.

In his notebook, Graham made explicit the connection between capital-

ism and physiological stress. In a section on "Mental Excitement," he
recorded what amounts to a paradigm of the way that life in the marketplace could pervert a man's dietary habits, and in this way bring him to
physical collapse. Graham chose the example of a businessman who is
forced to spend much of his time in an "auction room"—a perfect symbol
of the marketplace. A day in the auction room, Graham noted, leads
to a whole system of unpleasant sensations: "anxiety-fear-doubt—sus-
pense—excitement." By the close of the business day the tradesman
returns to his home in a state of complete "exhaustion." He has absolutely
"no appetite for dinner." But, in an effort to keep himself going, and
give himself the energy to return to work the next day, he turns to the battery of "artificial preparations" which a commercial society has "invented"
in order to "excite desire"—all the "spices, stimulants, and condiments"
of the modern kitchen. To be sure, these stimulants manage to arouse his
appetite (in fact, to overarouse it), but at the same time they intensify
his exahustion.[7] By turning to them, the businessman has reproduced in
his private life, in his pattern of consumption, the same destructive cycle
he is simultaneously experiencing in his public life in the auction house:
the cycle of stimulation . . . exhaustion . . . stimulation . . . and eventual
death.

Sylvester Graham was not the only American of his generation to
sense a connection between conditions in the marketplace and the conditions of personal experience. It is more than coincidence that terms such
as "panic" and "depression"—both words relating to emotional states—
were coming in the 1830s to be applied to the boom-bust economic cycles
generated in these years by emerging marketplace conditions. Jacksonian
economic reformers tended to speak of the new commercial economy as
"fevered," and Andrew Jackson himself attacked unnatural emissions of
paper money (the exact financial equivalents of artificial dietary stimulants). The year of the Great Panic, 1837, provided the economic cor-
relative to Graham's physiological analysis. It proved that the nation
needed to return to a state of serenity and subsistence, to follow the same
prescription Graham recommended for the hapless businessman who
worked in the auction house: wash in cold water, "sit down and rest,"
and "take a plain piece of stale bread or cracker and deliberately chew
it."[8]

For many middle-class Jacksonian men, it was the nuclear family, newly sentimentalized, that was coming (at least in theory) to perform this therapeutic function, to serve as the sole bastion of serenity in the heart of an otherwise frenetic world. For other Jacksonians, it was "nature" that performed this same function, or a new and softened form of Christianity. Along with these people, Sylvester Graham implicitly conceded that the world itself could not be changed—the auction house, for instance, would remain. (It is significant that Graham could not, or would not, make the simple suggestion that his businessman look for a less strenuous occupation.) Along with many other Jacksonians, Graham suggested that it was necessary to devise an oasis in the midst of this hectic world. He was unique only in that he located the oasis not in the family, not in "nature," not in religion, but within the individual human body. The physical organism itself was his proposed utopian retreat, his Walden Pond—an *inner* space where "decorum and sanctity reign" (to use Emerson's phrase) and no "calamity" can strike.[9]

In his *Lectures on the Science of Human Life,* Graham systematically expounded the underlying principles of physiology which made it possible for him to propose the radical idea that the human organism could be dissociated from the world around it. And it was here that Graham fastened most tenaciously on the work of the French physiologist Xavier Bichat—to whose vitalism, and particularly to whose distinction between "animal" and "organic" existence, we must turn again.

Bichat spoke of "animal" existence, in so many words, as life "in the world," and he spoke of "organic" existence as life "within the self."[10] This, of course, was just the kind of distinction that seemed best to serve Graham's larger purposes. But there was a problem here: Graham's larger purposes were not quite the same as Bichat's. After all, the French physician was a child of the Enlightenment who had written at the end of the eighteenth century, in a social and intellectual world somewhat different from that of Jacksonian America. Graham, therefore, was forced to be selective in what he took from Bichat and to ignore the implications of Bichat's ideas even as he employed the Frenchman's language.

When Bichat defined animal life as existence "in the world," and organic life as existence "within the self," he did so in order to emphasize the malleability and superiority of the one in contrast to the obvious limitations of the other. Animal life, Bichat wrote, was "susceptible of extension and perfection," whereas organic life was "unchangeably fixed to the limits Nature has assigned it." Since the essence of human nature was precisely its openendedness, it was therefore "by animal life that man is so great, so superior to the beings around him." Science, art, industry, commerce, society itself—everything by which man may distinguish himself from the brutes—was for Bichat the product of animal life. Organic life, on the other hand, was the seat of the primitive and uncontrollable passions, of everything subhuman in man's nature. (The relative valuation Bichat placed on animal and organic life is suggested by his insistence that murder is a criminal act only because of its destruction of animal life. It was on these grounds, for instance, that Bichat defended abortion: In killing the fetus, the French physician claimed, one destroyed a creature who only "lived" organically in the first place.)

The animal-organic distinction, as Bichat described it, was little more than a physiological version of the old distinction between head and heart—man's higher and lower natures. In fact, Bichat actually described life as a constant struggle within each individual between organic and animal impulses. Those men in whom the organic element is dominant, he argued, are passionate and impulsive: they are governed by "the gastric and pectoral organs." Those men in whom the animal element is dominant are governed, on the other hand, by "sensation, perception, and intelligence." The happiest person, Bichat concluded in fine eighteenth-century style, "is he who has the two lives in a sort of equilibrium."[11]

Graham seized on Bichat's distinction between organic and animal existence, and he accepted the anatomical and physiological theories by which Bichat distinguished the one from the other. But Graham came close to reversing the Frenchman's relative appraisal of the two systems. Graham was not convinced of the superiority of man over the brutes. After all, the developments Bichat lauded as humanity's greatest achievements—science, commerce, society—were for Graham at the root of man's moral and physiological degradation. Graham disparaged even reason itself, which led to those achievements. "Of all the animals which inhabit this beautiful sphere," Graham wrote in the Lecture on Chastity, ". . . proud, rational man is the only one who has degraded his nature, and, by his voluntary depravity, rendered this life a pilgrimage of pain."

For this reason Graham placed a higher value on those characteristics mankind shared with the lower animals than on those that were uniquely

human. Graham defended his preference with evidence Bichat himself
had provided—by citing, for example, the fact that organic life develops
at an earlier point in time than animal life, or that vital existence can
continue even when the senses, the voluntary muscles, and the brain itself have ceased to function. Graham made much of the notion that the
organic system could perform, if necessary, without the aid of the brain,
"all the functions immediately essential to animal and organic life";
whereas the animal system by itself could not survive for more than
"a single moment." There were many cases, Graham reported, in which
individuals had survived for extended periods of time "in a state of sus-
pended consciousness or animation." There were even cases in which
the organic nervous system took over the functions of a defective brain.

Graham denied that the brain was the source of the nervous energy
which sustained the vital processes. That source, he claimed, lay in the
organic nervous system—and especially in the semilunar ganglions and
the *solar plexus*. For Graham, the *solar plexus* was the "brain" of organic
life and the "general centre of action" to the whole body. The brain
itself, "instead of being a galvanic apparatus employed in generating the
nervous power or vital stimulus of the whole system, is appropriated
entirely to the intellectual powers and manifestations, and has little
more to do with the rest of the body than to depend on its general organic economy for its own sustenance."[12]

What is notable about Graham's emphasis on the autonomous viability
of organic life is the fact that it defined human existence in a wholly in-
ternalized manner. In effect it removed people from the environment—
animal life was "in the world"—or, more accurately, it made people's
own internal functions their only "natural" environment. Implicit in
this aspect of Graham's theory was the assumption that at no point
did individuals have to confront the outside world in order to survive.
They did not have to engage in science, art, industry, commerce, or in
society itself. They did not have even to think, move, or feel. They were
able to be wholly passive. They were able to remain—and this was a metaphor which was deeply rooted in physiological reality—in an Eden of
perpetual infancy.

But in the world as it had become, people were propelled out of the
sanctuary of their self-sufficient childhood and into the hostile environment of the world. Here the vitalistic theory that Graham borrowed from

Bichat provided him with a conceptual framework in which he could account for the hostility of the modern marketplace. That new order was represented by the "inorganic affinities" of chemical and physical law, which continuously threatened to overwhelm the tiny oasis of vitality struggling in their midst. Life was "a continued, antagonistic conflict between vitality . . . and the more primitive affinities of inorganic chemistry"; it was nothing more than "a temporary victory over the causes which induce death." The conditions of battle were weighted against the living organism, since by continually ingesting a portion of its environment in order to insure even temporary survival, it was forced literally to open its gates to the enemy. As Graham expressed it, the body "subsists on foreign substances, on materials extrinsic and separate from itself."

During infancy and childhood people were protected to a considerable degree from this danger, since the nourishment they consumed—mother's milk or home-baked bread—was of the safest and most soothing variety. (Indeed, this food was virtually the substance of the mother's body— literally in the one case, figuratively in the other.) But with the onset of adulthood came the loss of all this protection. A grown person faced the world on his own, and that world no longer took the benevolent form of his mother or the food she provided.[13]

It was only to provide some measure of purely internal protection to replace the lost external protection of childhood that the organism developed its system of animal life. The animal system, as Graham took every opportunity to point out, had no ultimate significance of its own. The sole purpose of the voluntary muscles, the five senses, even the brain itself, was to protect and preserve the integrity of the organic system, which alone was able to sustain life. (It was for this reason that Graham so often emphasized that the brain—mankind's most highly developed possession—was a mere animal organ.) The animal system functioned, in effect, as the organism's department of state, or perhaps as its department of defense. This role could be seen clearly in the voluntary muscles, which enabled the organism to avoid dangers by moving away from them, or, if necessary, to subdue them through the application of physical force. As for the brain, its role was simply to gauge the significance of impulses received by the five senses, and to issue appropriate commands to the muscles. The brain was the organ "through which the mind is acted on by the body, and in turn, acts on the body."

Finally, the purpose of the five senses was to provide the original indications of danger. Graham actually employed a set of military images when he discussed the senses. Speaking of the body as if it were a fortress or a nation whose borders were under siege, he referred to the sensory organs as the "sentinels" of the body. The nose, for instance, was an "olefactory sentinel . . . placed on the outposts of the vital domain," whose duty it was to warn the lungs and the alimentary canal about the presence of any element "unfriendly to life" in the atmosphere. When such an element thus betrayed its presence, the organism reacted with a characteristic withdrawal: it attempted "to suspend respiration for a very short time and to hasten from the offending cause."[14]

As the sentinels and protectors of the body, the muscles, brain, and senses—the animal system of life—had to respond sensitively and accurately to every impulse from the surrounding environment. A sensitive response was required so that not even the faintest of these potentially lethal signals would escape the body's notice, and an accurate one was needed so that the body could determine whether a given signal indicated danger. A sense of taste so "depraved" that it did not cause the body to reject (i.e., by gagging) such substances as alcohol, tobacco, or meat, clearly left the organism in an extremely vulnerable condition. It was far better for the animal system to overreact than to underreact to external stimuli. Thus an individual whose olefactory nerves were perfectly healthy would automatically respond with symptoms of headache, nervous discomfort, perspiration, fever, and chills upon breathing "air which is loaded with the perfumes of a garden of roses and other flowers; or the air of a room containing several pots of geranium." Indeed, Graham added in a curiously self-defeating footnote, "many individuals have died suddenly in consequence of inspiring the too powerful perfume of roses and other fragrant flowers accumulated in large quantities."[15]

In the newspapers of the 1830s Graham made a discovery that revealed to him the apotheosis of animal sensitivity. It was the story of a German youth named Caspar Hauser, who claimed to have been confined for unknown reasons "in a narrow, dark dungeon" from his early childhood until he was about seventeen. During this whole period, as Graham reported the tale, Hauser "was kept in a sitting posture with no other clothing than a shirt, and made to subsist on coarse, brown bread and water exclusively." Yet at the time of his release his body had developed with "remarkable symmetry and beauty," and furthermore the acuteness and power of his sight, hearing, smell, taste and touch, far exceeded anything of the kind ever before known in a human being." Graham reported his accomplishments in admiring detail: Hauser was unerringly able to determine the identity of colors in almost total darkness; he was able to distinguish different people in a crowd by the sound of their footsteps; and he was able to identify almost any plant at a distance by the smell of its leaves. "Indeed the power of all his senses seemed miraculous." Not only were Hauser's senses extraordinarily powerful, they were also unfailingly accurate barometers of danger: Hauser reacted with manifest abhorrence to even the faintest smell or taste of alcohol, meat, or spices, no matter how carefully these substances were hidden or disguised. At the same time, as Graham indicated, "all farinaceous preparations and proper fruits, very readily became agreeable to him."[16]

Through the operations of the animal system, then, a healthy body became totally sensitive to every impulse present in its immediate environment. But by the same token, through the operations of its organic system, such a body remained totally insensible to those impulses that originated within itself. The organic system, as Bichat had noted, was naturally devoid of animal sensibility. As Graham explained, a healthy individual did not have "the least consciousness of any internal organ," and if he were to feel such a consciousness, he could be "certain that something is wrong." To begin with, organic sensibility (in the form of hunger or lust, for example) indicated a waste of vital energy, much like a battery draining its current. Every individual, Graham noted, "comes into existence with a determinate amount of constitutional stamina—an unreplenishable fund of life"; and since "all vital action is necessarily attended with the expenditure of [this] vital power, [it] draws something from the ultimate and unreplenishable fund of life—and therefore, all excessive vital action—all intensity of vital action, increases the expenditure of vital power, and necessarily abbreviates the duration of life."

More immediately, organic sensibility blunted or "depraved" the animal senses. As Graham indicated even in the *Lecture on Chastity,* excessive lust could virtually destroy the sight, the smell, the taste, the hearing, and the touch; and as he insisted at length in the *Lectures on the Science of Human Life,* even what passes for "normal" sensitivity in these areas was only a shadow of the truly healthy condition exemplified by Caspar Hauser. Finally, organic sensibility diverted the attention of the individual away from its proper object—the external environment. An organism under constant danger of attack from without could scarcely afford to deal with rebellion from within, whether it took the form of disease or of need, discomfort or pleasure. In Graham's own metaphor, the ability of a nation to defend its borders was a direct function of its own domestic tranquility.[17]

But the greatest danger to which unnatural organic sensibility exposed an individual was the prospect that it would cause him to lose his precarious hold on objective reality—the reality of the world around him. It would cause him to mistake sensations which actually originated within his own body for sensations that seemed to originate in the environment. It would cause him, literally or figuratively, to hallucinate. Graham argued, for instance, that feelings of exaltation and despair (even those commonly induced by intense religious experience) the effects of a revival, for instance) were simply the products of physiological irritation. Such feelings had no more substance than those resulting from inebriation. Both conditions were substance than those resulting from inebriation, and both conditions were generated by the body itself—by the operations of a deranged organic system—and they indicated nothing about the real world. Graham drew a sharp distinction between the mental images which resulted from the actual sight of an object and those which resulted from memory or imagination—in other words, those with an internal origin. The former he referred to as "perceptions," and the latter as "conceptions." The two phenomena were absolutely incompatible: Graham insisted it was impossible "for the mind to have a distinct perception and conception at one and the same instant."

Conceptions, Graham argued, were generally false and misleading. Whether they took the form of waking fantasies, nocturnal dreams, drunken hallucinations, or the demons of insanity itself, they bore no relationship to external reality. All were the products of nervous irritation, and the differences among them were merely differences of degree. Insanity, in other words, was the result of a continual and intense dosage of the same dietary or sexual irregularity which in milder forms produced ordinary dreams and fantasies. But whether temporarily or permanently, the dreamer, the drunkard, and the madman were equally out of touch with the world around them—and equally unable to cope with that world.[18]

An effort to formulate a technique by which solitary individuals could insulate themselves from a constantly threatening world was at the core of the "science of human life." From virtually the beginning of his professional career, Graham dismissed the possibility that any traditional source of institutional guidance and authority—law, government, the Bible, church, school, or even family—could for any length of time effectively mediate between the individual and his environment. As early as his first published work, an 1829 sermon on Sunday schooling, Graham contended that "civil legislation may exhaust itself in adding statute to statute" without providing real control over human behavior. He repeated this claim, and enlarged on it, in the Lecture on Chastity: "To what avail," he asked, "are moral laws, and civil legislation, and philanthropic efforts" in the effort to help the human race?[19]

Along with other members of his generation—Ralph Waldo Emerson, for one, whose career paralleled Graham's—Graham maintained that the only legitimate and effective source of human order was to be discovered within man himself. As he wrote in the Lecture on Chastity, "moral and civil laws, so far as they are right and proper, are only the verbal forms of laws which are constitutionally established in our nature."[20]

Historically speaking, statements such as these marked the dramatic inversion of a long-held sense of the relationship between individuals and social institutions—an inversion that is apparent also in other areas of American thought during the 1830s. In an earlier day, it was assumed that individuals were naturally undependable and unstable; stability and order therefore had to be inherent in society itself. Men devised and nurtured a whole set of institutions—family, church, and "government"—to produce this order. Such institutions existed to insure that individuals would be subjected to the constant scrutiny of a wider community that might transcend the imperfections of the individuals who composed it. This way of looking at things is as evident in the social theory of the Founding Fathers at the end of the eighteenth century as it is in the social theory of the New England Puritans in the middle of the seventeenth. It was only during the 1830s that it was challenged—and, indeed, turned on its head. Now it was society itself and its institutions that were seen as the locus of instability, and the individual who was seen as the one potential source of order. A person had to become his own "community," his own agency of regulation. In place of scrutiny, control, and protection imposed (and guaranteed) from without, he had to impose these things upon himself.

But in contrast to the confidence that appeared to underlie Emerson's appeal to individual consciousness, Graham's reduction of ethics into hygiene was informed by a sense of urgency and desperation. The ideal type of "Grahamite man" looked upon an environment which took the form not of an Emersonian landscape but of a Melvilleian ocean—a hostile void. The ordinary mode in which he confronted this environment, likewise, was not as a "transparent eyeball" but as a beast in the jungle—a beast that combined the armor of a turtle with the sensitivity of a jackrabbit. Protected from without by virtue of his ability to perceive danger and avoid it, and secured from within by virtue of a regimen which minimized the demands of his own body, the Grahamite man stood ready to face the world unaided by any external source of strength. He was a solitary figure who had been forced to purchase his continued survival at the cost of much that in the eyes of both an earlier and a later age made him human.

The Grahamite man also was suggestively close to the figure of the archetypical Jacksonian in all his forms, from rural frontiersman to urban entrepreneur. If his protective posture denied him access to a significant range of emotions, it simultaneously permitted him to release an enormous amount of directed energy into the world. Grahamite man, Ahab-like, might have failed badly at love or art, but he was apt to pursue his work with a single-minded determination. He was likely to be effective at the production of worldly goods. It was only as a consumer, and not as a producer, that he had rejected the marketplace. Seeing every man as a competitor, tackling every problem as if it concealed a conspiracy, resisting every indulgence as if it carried his doom, this Grahamite-Jacksonian creature inched his way through a world as atomized as himself. Yet his style, however constricted, was uniquely appropriate for a man, or a generation, that needed to create or to sustain the characteristic posture which a later generation would extol—and a still later one would condemn—as bourgeois.[21]

But if Grahamite theory helped lead to the creation of the bourgeois character, it did so in an unintended and roundabout fashion. That character type emerged out of a volatile mix of anxiety and nostalgia. The triumph of the new order was indirectly hastened by the sentimentalization of the old one. What can be called the physiology of subsistence was born, much like the religion of nature or the cult of domesticity, in an effort to resist and deny the reality of marketplace capitalism. But, like them, it too ended by reinforcing that reality.

NOTES

1. Sylvester Graham, *Lectures on the Science of Human Life*, 2 vols. (Boston, 1839), 2: 485.

2. Ibid., 2: 327, 492, 496.

3. Ibid., 2: 337-338.

4. In much the same fashion, Graham insisted in his *Lecture on Chastity* that vegetarians are capable of having "so subdued their sexual propensity" as to permit them to "abstain from connubial commerce . . . for several months in succession, without the least inconvenience." Sylvester Graham, *A Lecture to Young Men, on Chastity, intended also for the serious consideration of parents and guardians* (Providence, 1834).

5. Graham, *Science*, 2: 537.

6. Sylvester Graham, unpublished lecture notes (1831-1847), American Antiquarian Society, pp. 82, 283; Graham, *Science*, 1: 478-485.

7. Graham, lecture notes, p. 377.

8. Ibid.

9. Ralph Waldo Emerson, "Nature," in Reginald L. Cook, ed., *R. W. Emerson, Selected Prose and Poetry* (New York, 1950), p. 6. It is no coincidence that Thoreau, who moved to Walden Pond in 1845 in order to live "deliberately" and thereby to avoid "desperation," adopted something close to Graham's regimen of temperance, vegetarianism, sexual abstinence, and (above all) minimal consumption. See Henry David Thoreau, *Walden* (1854), esp. chapters 1, 2, and (on sexuality) 11.

10. Xavier Bichat, *Physiological Researches upon Life and Death* (Philadelphia, 1809), pp. 2-3, 7.

11. Ibid., pp. 43-47, 63-64, 103-109.

12. Graham, *Science*, 1: 121-157.

13. Graham, *A Lecture on Epidemic Diseases Generally, and Particularly the Spasmodic Cholera, delivered in . . . New York, March, 1832* (New York, 1833), p. 5; *Science*, 1: 490. The organism was forced to engage its environment to insure not only its survival as an individual (through nutrition), but also its survival as a species (through reproduction). It is no coincidence that Graham devoted the major part of his career to an analysis of these two phenomena.

14. Graham, *Science*, 1: 493-495.

15. Ibid.

16. Graham, *Science*, 2: 287-299. Graham took pains to argue that Caspar Hauser's remarkable abilities were more the product of his diet of bran bread and water than of his confinement in a dark and stimulus-free room. It is nevertheless interesting that Hauser's dungeon environment (diet included) was in several ways a version of the extended infancy and childhood for which Graham argued on several occasions: the walls of his cell both literally and symbolically secluded him from the hostile incursions of the outside world, in the form both of other people and of visual, aural, and olefactory stimulation. As Graham put it, Hauser was protected "from the light and from the ordinary influences of society" (pp. 288-289). What made this story such a perfect case for Graham was the fact that if prison protected

Hauser by providing an almost total nonenvironment, the youth was equally protected after his release by virtue of the animal sensitivity with which his years in prison had endowed him.

17. Graham, *Chastity*, pp. 115-117; *Science*, 1: 190, 491-588.

18. Graham, *Science*, 1: 386-410.

19. Sylvester Graham, "They Kingdom Come, A discourse on the importance of infant and Sunday Schools, delivered at Philadelphia, Dec. 13, 1829" (Philadelphia, 1831), pp. 24-25; Graham, *Chastity*, pp. 63, 165-169. See also *Genius of Temperance*, June 29, 1831.

20. The implications of statements such as these further reveal Graham's intellectual kinship with other types of antebellum reformers—especially the abolitionists. If moral and civil laws must reflect internal physiological "laws" in order to be considered "right and proper," it follows that laws that violate our physiological nature are improper. Not only is this idea analogous to the "higher law" argument invoked by antislavery orators, but, as Ronald G. Walters has pointed out, it actually formed a key element in the abolitionist critique of slave society. To middle-class northerners like Theodore Dwight Weld, the licentiousness fostered by the sexual availability of slaves was a prime index of the unnaturalness of southern institutions. In Weld's case, as in others, the ideological bridge between sensuality and unnaturalness was provided by Grahamite physiology. (Weld himself and his wife Angelina Grimké were practicing Grahamites.) According to Walters, the sharp contrast between reformers' self-imposed sexual restraint and the opportunities open to slaveholders gave the antislavery crusade most of its emotional impact. See Ronald G. Walters, "The Erotic South: Civilization and Sexuality in American Abolitionism," *American Quarterly* 25 (1973): 177-201.

21. In his *Horrors of the Half-Known Life* (New York, 1976), Graham Barker-Benfield has similarly argued that Jacksonian hygiene needs to be seen as an attempt to guide bourgeois males through the hostile, competitive world of commercial capitalism (see pp. 23-36). I have already expressed some doubt about his further assertion—that the main way these hygienic theories *functioned* was both to deny female sexuality and to establish male control of the female reproductive system. If Graham's ideas, as I believe, are representative of his era, they suggest additional grounds on which to dissociate Barker-Benfield's conclusions from one another. First, Graham's obvious need to integrate his sexual notions into a comprehensive world view implies a broader function for his version of the "spermatic economy" than the rationalizing of sex roles and the bolstering of sexual identity. Second, Graham's sexual theories could be and were used to undermine men's control over their wives—as the American career of Mary Gove Nichols indicates.

9. THE GRAHAM SYSTEM AT WORK

One of the most striking facts about the Graham System was that, for many people, it worked. Thousands of people in the 1830s attended Sylvester Graham's lectures, read his books, and, for a time at least, changed their lives. They did so, if their own testimony is to be believed, not in order to enter the emergent middle class, but for a simpler and even more pressing reason: They were sick, and they wished to become well.

Immediately after Graham took his lecture series outside the Philadelphia area, he began to receive testimonial letters from men who reported that their lives had been radically improved by changing their habits in the way Graham was suggesting. In 1833 Graham published some of the letters in a small volume titled *The Aesculapian Tablets of the Nineteenth Century.* Later in the decade other letters of a similar nature were published in the *Graham Journal of Health and Longevity,* a periodical published by Grahamites in the Boston area. The collective picture that emerges from these letters is one of fear, alienation, and the inability to cope with life—what one correspondent referred to as "a general debility of body and mind." Physical and emotional symptoms are inextricably linked in the testimonial letters, "spasmodic cough" with "nervous irritability," and "flatulency and . . . diarrhoea" with "low spirits, peevish, timid, and melancholy, bordering on insanity."[1]

Take this report, written to Sylvester Graham in 1833 by a worker in a suburban New York City cotton mill:

> Besides my intense and unbroken melancholy, and dark despondency of spirits, I was afflicted with distressing dizziness of the head, blindness, staggering, reeling, weakness, stammering and catching of voice.

Excessive irritability and weakness of stomach; no appetite. Extremely nervous; twitching of the different parts of my face; eyes very dull, weak and watery; deafness, and absence of mind; great aversion to company; sometimes severe headache; dull, stupid, and sluggish; after eating restless, uneasiness, very sleepy; yellowness of the skin and eyes; at times very sour stomach; sometimes sore throat, and raising of blood, depression of the chest and difficulty of breathing; wild appearance out of the eyes; internal soreness at the lower part of the stomach or chest; extreme fretfulness or peevishness; starting or jumping at any sudden noise or touch; memory very poor, and frequent alienation of mind; weariness of life; great desire for seclusion, or retirement; and often a reluctance to speak when spoken to; considerable fever at intervals; occasionally raising from the lungs hard, tough, green, putrid lumps of matter; easily irritated, and passions ungovernable. . . .[2]

Or this one, written the same year by a thirty-nine-year-old carpenter living in New York City who suffered from curious and continual "paroxysms" that attacked body and mind:

I became excessively nervous, so that I was continually full of apprehensions of danger, afraid of every thing, and starting with alarm at almost every thing. If any thing came upon me suddenly, it affected me very much. . . . I often became so much embarrassed and confused, that I would lose the power of speech; and frequently, when in conversation, I used suddenly to lose my thoughts in the midst of a sentence, and totally forgot what I was talking about. . . . When out from home, I was often attacked with these turns in the street, and became so much confused and bewildered, that it was with great difficulty that I could find the way to my house. . . .[3]

Some of these symptoms point to "real" disease; others to emotional strain. But the single unavoidable fact is that all the symptoms seemed to disappear (or at least to become tolerable) when the two men adopted the Graham System. Whatever it was that ailed the hundreds of people who composed such testimonials during the 1830s, it was something they were able to assuage by a drastic and repressive change in their dietary and sexual practices.

How did it work? What did the Graham System do for them that more orthodox remedies—prescribed by the regular physicians these people had invariably consulted at an earlier time—did not do? To begin with, the Graham System organized their symptoms into a coherent syndrome with a single comprehensible cause, and it was a cause that could be remedied. According to the "Science of Human Life," their ailments did not originate in the confusing array of external circumstances over which they had no control, but rather in that single area of their lives for which they could assume total responsibility: the ordinary daily routine of private habit. If these sick men could not be in command of the world around them, they could at least take charge of their own bodies.

The practical message of the Graham System, then, was that the very routine of daily existence, which until recently had been regulated by the community or dictated by the natural rhythms of rural life, was actually a matter of considerable urgency. The little things that scarcely seemed worthy of conscious notice—when to get up in the morning and go to bed at night, what to eat and how much, how often and in what way to obtain sexual release—had to be subjected to the same degree of intense scrutiny traditionally reserved for matters of public behavior. For a person to achieve a state of well-being, according to the Graham System, his daily life had to be lifted from the trough of unexamined "routine" to the level of *consciousness*—and thereby to the level of conscious control—and become, in the term used by everyone connected with this movement, a "regimen." Before the 1830s the word *regimen* had referred to the rules to be followed in overcoming disease; now it came, rather abruptly, to refer to daily life itself.

Routine become "regimen": this was the core of the Graham System. Nowhere was the process better revealed than in its earliest institutionalized setting, the so-called Graham Boardinghouses. The first of these boardinghouses was established as early as 1833 in New York City (in Graham's name, though not under his direction) by converting a private residence into a temperance hotel, where men (no women were allowed) could temporarily stay for a "cold-turkey" Grahamite cure. The boardinghouse regulated every aspect of private live. The vegetarian meals, prepared only twice a day, and at precise hours, were small and nonstimulating, and they were served without spices or condiments. Drink consisted of cold water. The hours of arising and retiring were regulated just as carefully: a bell rang every morning "precisely at 5 o'clock (6 o'clock in the winter), on the principle that "one hour is necessary for bathing and exercise before breakfast." At night, doors were locked and lights doused at "precisely" 10 o'clock, and clients were not given keys. During the day, of course, the residents—they included Horace Greeley and William Lloyd Garrison—were free to go about their ordinary business affairs.[4]

The Graham System spread rather rapidly in the mid-1830s. A second boardinghouse was established at Boston in 1836 under the direction of a man named David Cambell, who had been active as a Garrisonian abolitionist earlier in the decade. In addition to managing the boardinghouse, Cambell edited the *Graham Journal of Health and Longevity* for the three years it was published, between 1837 and 1839. In the latter year he abandoned both of his projects and moved to Oberlin, Ohio, where Charles G. Finney had asked him to become the "steward" at Oberlin College. Oberlin had forbidden the consumption of "tea and coffee, highly seasoned meats, rich pastries and all unwholesome [sic] and expensive foods" in the year in which it was established, 1832. An "Oberlin Physiological Society" had been founded by both students and staff in 1838—Finney himself served on its executive committee—and physiology was made a required course at the college. From the time Cambell assumed his duties as steward, no more animal food was served in commons—previously there had been an "elective" meat table—and the menu was prepared in strict accordance with the principles of the Graham system. Cambell even planned to establish a Graham boardinghouse for the use of the Oberlin community, but this project apparently fell through.[5]

Before Cambell moved to Oberlin, he had been an officer of the American Physiological Society, an organization founded in Boston in 1837 along Grahamite lines. Graham himself lectured to the group a number of times, and one of its principal functions was the dissemination of information about the Graham System. It also sponsored the establishment of a local "Graham store."[6]

One hundred and twenty-four men joined the American Physiological Society when it was organized in 1837. (Their names are listed at the end of the group's constitution.) An examination of Boston's city directories and property valuation lists, federal census schedules, and Massachusetts vital records, offers information about many of these men—information that can help to increase our understanding of the Graham System and the nature of its appeal in Jacksonian America.[7]

Most of the members seem to have been young men. Of forty-nine members whose exact ages can be determined, thirty-seven of them (or 76 percent) were between the ages of twenty-five and forty at the time they joined. These were men who had only recently established their families and their jobs.

Most of them seem to have been born in the small towns of rural New England. Of the thirty-six men whose exact place of birth can be determined, twenty-nine (or 81 percent) were born in small rural communities: twelve in western or southern Massachusetts, ten in New Hampshire, and seven scattered among Maine, Vermont, Connecticut, and upstate New York. Of the remaining seven, four were born in towns near Boston, and three were immigrants from Britain. Not one of the thirty-six was a native of Boston proper; they were all newcomers to the city in which they worked. These were men who literally had moved into the world of the marketplace.

The occupations of these men are particularly interesting. Virtually all of them were either skilled artisans or tradesmen. Of the eighty-four members whose occupations have been determined, all except three or four fit this description. Six of them were "housewrights" (i.e., house builders); five were piano makers; four were grocers, and another four were listed simply as "merchants." There were three each of cabinet makers, book-binders, and machinists as well as assorted dealers of dry goods, hats, confectionaries, stoves, wooden wares, and other household products. Conspicuously absent from the American Physiological Society were the two ends of the economic scale: unskilled laborers and professional men. There were no lawyers, no bankers, no physicians, no commission merchants, no public figures—in short, no members of Boston's elite.

The middling status of these men is confirmed by economic data. In or about 1837, eighty-five of the members were listed as owners of property in Boston—real property, personal property, or both. The median holding for the eighty-five men was exactly $1,000. Forty-five of them (or 52 percent) owned $1,000 or less. (Most of these, thirty-two, owned no more than $400.) Another twenty-four members (or 28 percent of the total) owned between $1,000 and $5,000. The remaining seventeen (the wealthiest 20 percent of the group) owned more than $5,000.

These, then, were men who were neither rich nor (in general) very poor, neither outside the marketplace nor secure in their position within it. The housewrights and the piano makers (two modal occupations among the membership) were typical. The construction of houses was a specialized occupation that had developed out of carpentry, and the construction of pianos was a specialized outgrowth of cabinet-making. Both were traditional artisan skills that probably had led most of these eleven men to their careers in Boston. Furthermore, by the 1830s both houses and pianos were rapidly being transformed from handcrafted, customized items into mass-produced commodities in highly competitive markets.[8]

One of the five piano makers, a man named Edwin Brown, moved to Boston shortly before 1832 and worked as a cabinet maker until 1834; but the next year, when twenty-nine years old, he opened a piano company in partnership with another man who apparently provided the capital. In 1838, the year after he joined the American Physiological Society, Brown patented a method for using the soft-pedal to dampen the piano's strings without shifting the inner mechanism of the instrument. Although he was living in a decade of the most rapid technological development in the history of the piano industry and successfully participating in it, Brown felt unhappy about himself, as his membership in the American Physiological Society suggests.[9] It is tempting to imagine that the Graham System, with its dependable routine and its radical rejection of marketplace values, gave him a way of dealing with the hectic and unfamiliar world on which his prosperity depended. Through the Graham System, he could remain fully engaged with the productive demands of his work, but at the same time persuade himself that he lived somewhere else, in an inner world of serenity and subsistence.

The men who joined the American Physiological Society seemed, at least by one important touchstone, to achieve a real degree of stability in their lives. Of the thirty-two members of the society whose place of residence at the time of their death can be determined, twenty-nine (or 91 percent) of them were still living within fifteen miles of Boston, and eighteen of these (or 56 percent of the total) were residents of Boston itself—a remarkably high rate of geographical persistence for such a mobile period.[10]

Sylvester Graham also achieved geographic stability in the last dozen years of his life, but, unlike many of his followers, he did so at the cost of his active career. He abandoned the lecture circuit when he bought his house in Northampton in 1839—the only house he ever owned. Graham never did manage to find the inner serenity he praised with such fervor.

After his death in 1851, one of Graham's followers described him as a man who was able to "see truth clearly, and yet not have the self-government to practice it." Graham's own wife adamantly opposed his strictures, and she subjected him to the constant temptations of a "table luxuriously spread" with forbidden food and drink. Graham openly acknowledged to his friends that he often succumbed to at least this one of his wife's temptations and that he often did "violence to his own doctrines."[11]

In addition to violating his own physiological rules, Graham betrayed himself economically by becoming ensnared in the tentacles of the capitalist marketplace. During the 1840s he invested most of his savings in railroad and canal stock at an inflated price based on the misrepresentations of the company. He claimed to have lost over $5,000 by 1851. In that year Graham's health was failing rapidly, and he blamed his decline not on dietary irregularity but on the "pecuniary embarrassments" that had led to an "excessive and even violent and protracted overworking of both my mind and body." His investments in the market, he wrote, had caused him to become an "utter wreck." The physician who examined Graham at about this time was unable to find any evidence of serious organic disease, and attributed his problems to the "somewhat irregular life" he had been leading.[12] Four months later, Sylvester Graham was dead at the age of fifty-seven.

Characteristically enough, Graham never joined the American Physiological Society. The man who helped him set it up, and who served as president of the society during its three-year existence (along with a number of other Grahamite organizations, it folded in 1839), was William Andrus Alcott (1798-1859), a physician, teacher, and writer whose hygienic principles were even more extreme than Graham's. (Alcott's recipe for coarse bread did not include any leavening agent—yeast, too, turned out to be a stimulant—and he believed that all liquid, even water, was unnecessary, and that thirst itself was an unnatural appetite.)

An enormously prolific and versatile writer, Alcott gained what Graham lost in personal influence during the late 1830s, and tracts like his *Vegetable Diet* (1838), *Tea and Coffee* (1839), *The Use of Tobacco* (1844), and *The Teacher of Health* (1843) reached enthusiastic audiences. Like Graham, Alcott treated sexual hygiene as a significant factor in general health. He included a long chapter on sexual abuses in *The Young Man's Guide* (1833), one of the earliest of his books and probably the most popular. Later in his career, titles such as *The Young Woman's Book of Health* (1850) and *Lectures on Life and Health* (1853) contained large chunks of sexual material. Alcott's major contribution to the genre, however, was *The Physiology of Marriage* (1856), a book he published anonymously—"by an old physician," the title page read—and which could almost have come from Graham's pen. It was followed the next year by a companion volume, *Moral Philosophy of Courtship and Marriage,* and Alcott apparently intended to pursue the subject still further at the time of his death in 1859.[13]

The principles of Grahamism reached an even wider and more heterogeneous public during the 1840s through a pair of connected reform movements: phrenology and the water-cure. The first of these, phrenology, originated at the beginning of the nineteenth century with the work of two Austrian physicians, Franz Joseph Gall and Johann Gaspar Spurzheim, and had been transmitted to America during the 1830s by Spurzheim himself and by a Scottish lawyer named George Combe. The theory was popularized in the following decade by a group of "practical phrenologists" who traversed the country delivering lectures and holding demonstrations. Phrenologists believed the diverse elements which made up individual character, temperament and ability—there were thirty-seven of them in all, according to Spurzheim, with labels including "combativeness," "approbativeness," and "philoprogenitiveness" (love of one's children)—were each controlled by a different, and definable, area of the brain. This rule applied both to the intellectual faculties and to the physical "propensities."[14]

Thus sexual desire (or "amativeness," as it was called) originated not in the genital organs but in a particular region of the brain—specifically, in the cerebellum. (Phrenologists felt that this particular discovery was extremely important: in 1838 George Combe published a collection of essays by Gall and others which claimed to provide unanswerable proof that the cerebellum was the true seat of lust.)[15]

To be sure, phrenology implied a theory of physiological process somewhat different from that articulated by Graham, and Graham was sufficiently aware of the difference to question the new science in his *Lectures.*[16] Nevertheless, many people, especially in America, believed that the two approaches were by no means incompatible, and "practical phrenologists" such as Orson S. Fowler (1809-1887) combined them enthusiastically.

(So, for that matter, did other, less likely, individuals: by the end of his life François Broussais had become the most prominent phrenologist in France.)[17]

Fowler, who had encountered phrenology as a student at Amherst College early in the 1830s, was confident that it was actually reinforced by "physiology" (as he termed the Graham System and its theoretical underpinnings), and that the two systems were most effectively employed in combination. This belief formed the structure of many of Fowler's books: temperance, for instance, was "founded on phrenology and physiology," as one of Fowler's titles put it. In the words of another title, "phrenology and physiology [should be] applied to man's social relations" or applied, again, "to the selection of a suitable companion for life."[18]

In these works, in the columns of his *American Phrenological Journal*, and in the lectures delivered on his tours, Fowler spoke unequivocally against the use of animal food and the usual catalogue of stimulants. One of his books, *Physiology, Animal and Mental* (1847), amounted to a phrenological paraphrase of the *Lectures on the Science of Human Life*. Employing Graham's vitalism, and adapting his analysis of the nervous system to the requirements of phrenology, Fowler included long sections on anatomy, physiology, health and disease, and diet—with special emphasis on the correct preparation of bread from unbolted flour, and a long section in defense of vegetable diet. As Fowler saw it, animal food and other stimulants tended to inflame that area of the brain—the area toward its base—which controlled the physical drives and emotions, or the "propensities," as they were called. ("Animal food . . . inflames Destructiveness, and renders it morbid as well as large," he wrote in a characteristic statement.)[19]

Fowler extended his analysis to the sexual "propensity" in a series of books, including one on *Amativeness* (ca. 1843) in which he warned about the dangers of "excessive and perverted sexuality" (dangers that included promiscuity, "matrimonial excess," and "self-abuse"); another on *Love and Parentage* (ca. 1843) in which he provided "important directions and suggestions to lovers and the married concerning the strongest ties and the most momentous relations of life"; and a third on *Maternity* (1848) in which he warned prospective mothers against any sexual excitement during their pregnancy or during the period of nursing that followed it—a period which was to last, according to Fowler, for at least two years.[20]

These books and others were publicized by Fowler and his associates in the course of their lecture tours. After lecturing, they would perform phrenological analyses of the members of the audience (analyses that really amounted to primitive aptitude tests). The books themselves invariably were printed by the firm of Fowlers and Wells, a New York publishing house formed by Orson Fowler, his brother Lorenzo, and Samuel R. Wells. Fowlers and Wells published a diversified list of books, and for two decades the firm served as the most important publicity channel for most of the latest discoveries in the field of popular science. A typical Fowlers and Wells advertisement was literally a catalogue of scientific reform, including phrenology, hygiene, vegetarianism, mesmerism, spiritualism, and (most especially) the water-cure.

It was in the movement for the water-cure (or "hydropathy," as it was commonly known) that the principles of Grahamism left what was perhaps their clearest legacy. As it had been developed in the 1820s by an Austrian named Vincent Priessnitz, the water-cure was simply a therapeutic system based on the external application of cold water to different parts of the body. (The application was made in a variety of ways—showers, baths, wet-packs, etc.) Hydropathists claimed that when these "natural" techniques were applied properly, they could effectively cure a number of ailments. When the system was popularized in America during the mid-1840s, however, it underwent the same transformation that had already affected American phrenology: instead of remaining in its pure form, the water-cure was superimposed on a well-formulated theory of Grahamite physiology and regimen.

The first important American hydropath, a man named Joel Shew (1816-1855), advocated a therapeutic system which emphasized exercise and an extreme version of the Graham diet as firmly as it did the water treatment itself.[21] The American Hydropathic Society, which Shew helped to organize in 1849 (along with Russell Thacher Trall and Samuel Wells) was replaced the following year by the American Hygienic and Hydropathic Society, which promised to disseminate "those physiological principles which are usually comprised under the term HYGIENE." Finally, all reference to water treatment was dropped in 1859, when the Hydropathic Society was in turn superseded by the National Health Organization.[22]

Russell Thacher Trall (1812-1877), who succeeded Shew late in the 1840s as the most prominent hydropathic physician in America, came to the water-cure from the temperance movement. (He had spent some years as editor of a Washingtonian periodical in Albany.) In 1849, when his reputation as a hydropathist was already fully secure, Trall and Wells helped organize the American Anti-Tobacco Society, and for a time he served as its president.[23] The following year, once again in company with the ubiquitous Wells, Trall was a moving spirit in the formation of the American Vegetarian Society—William A. Alcott became its president— and he was made a member of the society's executive committee. When the official publication of the society, the *American Vegetarian and Health Journal,* folded in 1854, Trall agreed to reserve for the organization's exclusive use two full pages in each issue of his own magazine, the *Water-Cure Journal* (which was itself published and subsidized by Fowlers and Wells). In 1855 the Vegetarian Society held its annual meeting—attended by Lucy Stone, Amelia Bloomer, Susan B. Anthony, and Horace Greeley—at Trall's hydropathic establishment in New York City.

The link between Grahamism and hydropathy became strikingly symbolized in 1845 when David Cambell, the former manager of the Graham boardinghouse in Boston and steward at Oberlin College, became general manager of Joel Shew's water-cure at New Lebanon Springs in upstate New York. Cambell remained in this position for ten years— a long tenure in the rapidly-shifting patterns of reform life in Jacksonian America. The Graham System had finally established a secure institutional base.[24]

The water-cure of the 1840s and 1850s was, in fact, a direct successor to the Graham boardinghouse of the 1830s. Trall's Hydropathic and Hygienic Institute, for example—an elaborate building which contained not only sleeping, dining and bathing facilities but also public rooms and a gymnasium—imposed a familiarly strict routine on the lives of its residents: meals were served, and baths taken, only at specified hours, and the building was locked for the night promptly at ten o'clock. House rules enjoined the use of tobacco or alcohol as well as "all lounging on the sofas." Besides providing its residents with water-treatment, proper diet, and a well-ordered existence, the Institute performed a variety of additional functions: it manufactured "all kinds of farinaceous preparations," including "pure and proper articles of wheaten grits, hominy, oatmeal, farina, crackers, etc."; and it provided this food even to those who did not care to take the water treatment but who wished to employ "the dietary of the institution." By the early 1860s Trall was selling Graham flour and other health foods for cash over the counter.[25] These probably included the first commercial versions of the modern Graham Cracker.

Trall was also quick to sense the expanding market for advice about sexual hygiene. He included such advice in his first important book, *The Hydropathic Encyclopedia* (1851), and during the following years he produced a number of works devoted exclusively to the subject—beginning with *Home Treatment for Sexual Abuses* (1853), subtitled "a practical treatise on the nature and causes of excessive and unnatural indulgence," continuing with *Nervous Debility* and *Pathology of the Reproductive Organs* (both of these in 1861), and concluding with *Sexual Physiology* (1864), a popular work that went through several editions. As Trall indicated in these books, the physicians in attendance at his hydropathic institute were ready to interview and treat persons of either sex who suffered from sexual maladies of any kind. He also suggested that these maladies, more often than not, were the result of sexual abuse.[26]

Like Trall, other hydropathic physicians catered to the demand for both health food and sexual advice.[27] One of these was James Caleb Jackson (1814-1895), a Garrisonian abolitionist during the 1830s, who in 1859 established a water-cure near Dansville, a rural community in upstate New York. To create a domestic, almost communitarian, aura for his Dansville establishment, Jackson named it "Our Home on the Hillside." He provided (in addition to the usual hydropathic and hygienic facilities) a variety of recreational and educational activities, including theater, concerts, outings and lectures—along with accommodations for guests who did not desire to receive treatment. "Our Home on the Hillside" was as much a resort as a sanitarium. Jackson advertised the place with an array of promotional literature, along with the usual vegetarian and temperance tracts ("Flesh as Food for Man," "How to Cure Drunkards," "Tobacco and Its Effect") and several longer works on sexual hygiene (*Hints on the Reproductive Organs,* published in 1853 and *The Sexual Organism and Its Healthy Management,* published in 1861). As a sideline, Jackson manufactured and marketed a variety of Grahamite health foods. At one point early in the 1860s while he was searching for a food with all the therapeutic properties of Graham bread but that could be packaged and preserved for an indefinite period, Jackson developed a product which he called "Granula"—a mixture of Graham flour and water baked and pressed into thin sheets, broken up, ground into bite-sized pieces, and finally baked again.[28]

"Granula" was the first cold breakfast cereal. Jackson attempted to market it, but with little success. The project might never have been revived except for the fact that a family of Seventh-Day Adventists from Battle Creek, Michigan, visited "Our Home" for a time during 1864 in order to consult with Jackson and learn his methods.

Seventh-Day Adventism had developed out of the Millerite religious crusade of the early 1840s. From its earliest years influential members of the sect advocated vegetarian diet and other Grahamite views. The group of Adventists that visited "Our Home on the Hillside" in 1864 was led by a "prophetess" named Ellen White, whose periodic religious visions were accepted by her fellow Adventists as divinely inspired. In one of these visions, Mrs. White had received a message about the ill effects of masturbation, a message that caused her to publish a book on the subject in 1864: *An Appeal to Mothers: The Great Cause of the Physical, Mental, and Moral Ruin of Many of the Children of Our Time.* (This book expounded Grahamite theories of sexuality and vegetarian diet, and quoted passages from Graham himself, Orson S. Fowler, Mary Gove Nichols—whom we shall discuss further in the next chapter—and James Caleb Jackson.)[29] Presumably it was her newly-honed interest in sexuality, diet, and the water-cure, that led Mrs. White and her family to visit Jackson in September 1864.

Less than a year later, in August 1865, Ellen White and her family revisited "Our Home on the Hillside" for a more urgent reason: her husband had been stricken with a severe case of paralysis, and she hoped that James Caleb Jackson's hydropathic regimen would cure him. When he failed to recover, Ellen White blamed only the peripheral features of Jackson's establishment—its social frivolity and religious unorthodoxy—while retaining her faith in its physiological premises. She returned to Battle Creek convinced that the vegetarian and hydropathic regimen practiced in Dansville needed only an infusion of Adventist principles in order to become truly therapeutic. At Christmas 1865, Ellen White received a divine vision instructing her to put these principles into practice by founding an Adventist health reform facility. Many of the faithful responded to her call with generous contributions, and the newly-built Western Health Reform Institute was opened in September 1866.[30]

After an initial period of success, Ellen White's Western Health Reform

Institute faltered, largely because of disputes within the Adventist leadership over its direction. But it experienced a resurgence after 1876, the year that John Harvey Kellogg, then twenty-four years old, was named its superintendent. Kellogg (1852-1943), a protégé and friend of the White family, had been sent to learn hydropathic medicine at the school operated by Russell Thacher Trall in New York City, and he had been able to convince the reluctant Whites to subsidize him while he supplemented his training under Trall with eduation at more conventional "allopathic" medical schools, from one of which he received a medical degree in 1875. Upon assuming leadership of the Western Health Reform Institute the next year, Kellogg renounced narrow medical sectarianism and declared his desire to transform the institute into a large-scale, popular, and scientifically respectable establishment. As a first step toward that end, in 1877 he gave it a new name: the Battle Creek Sanitarium.[31]

But Kellogg's notion of scientific respectability meant only that he played down Adventist religious ideas, not that he abandoned the principles of Grahamism and hydropathic medicine. As his literary output suggests (in volume it surpassed that of both Trall and Jackson), those principles remained at the heart of his system, and they were put into practice at the "San," as his increasingly-popular Institute came to be known. Kellogg's first book, published in 1877, was an antimasturbation work titled *Plain Facts about Sexual Life;* and he later wrote works including *The Natural Diet of Man; The Physical, Moral and Social Effects of Alcoholic Poison;* and *Tobaccoism, or How Tobacco Kills.* To the end of his long career, Kellogg saw himself as a crusader against "the artificial conditions of civilized life."[32]

In 1878, two years after he took over the Battle Creek Sanitarium, Kellogg began to market a Grahamite cereal he called "Granola." James Caleb Jackson, who had patented his "Granula," immediately took him to court, but Kellogg went on to develop newer and better cereals. By 1900 he had come out with a primitive version of what soon became known as "cornflakes," and a short time later the modern breakfast cereal industry began to emerge.[33] The industry is still with us—although the consumption of cold breakfast cereals has remained a uniquely American habit. Along with the Battle Creek Sanitarium and other institutions like it, the breakfast cereal industry was perhaps the final institutionalization of the principles Sylvester Graham had first articulated two genera-

tions earlier. The Graham System itself, born as a physiology of subsistence, had been transformed into an industrialized commercial product.

NOTES

1. Letter of Nathaniel Perry, in *Graham Journal of Health and Longevity*
1 (1837): 3.
2. Letter of Charles Lewis, in Sylvester Graham, ed., *The Aesculapian
Tablets of the Nineteenth Century* (Providence, 1834), p. 63.
3. Letter of James Little, ibid., p. 82. Intriguing fictional parallels to these
symptoms, from the same period, can be found in the works of several writers
including Nathaniel Hawthorne (Arthur Dimmesdale in *The Scarlet Letter*,
Roderick Elliston in "Egotism, or The Bosom Serpent") and Edgar Allen Poe
("The Black Cat" and "The Tell-Tale Heart").
4. *Graham Journal*, p. 47; William B. Walker, "The Health Reform Movement in the United States, 1830-1870" (Ph.D. diss., Johns Hopkins University, 1955),
p. 40; Thomas H. Le Duc, "Grahamites and Garrisonites," *New York History*
20 (1939): 189-191.
5. Robert S. Fletcher, "Bread and Doctrine at Oberlin," *Ohio State
Archaeological and Historical Quarterly* 49 (1940): 58-67; Walker, "Health
Reform," pp. 134-139. Graham clubs were also established at other colleges,
including Lane Seminary in Cincinnati, Wesleyan University, and Williams
College (Walker, "Health Reform," pp. 135-136). Grahamism seemed to have
its greatest appeal in the newer, rural colleges.
6. H. E. Hoff and J. F. Fulton, "Centenary of the American Physiological
Society, Founded at Boston by William Andrus Alcott and Sylvester Graham,"
Bulletin of the Institute of the History of Medicine 5 (1937): 687-722; Walker,
"Health Reform," pp. 113-118. Four branch units of the Society were established
in New England and New York City.
7. Except as otherwise noted, the information in the next seven paragraphs is
derived from the following sources: Hoff and Fulton, "Centenary," pp. 731-733;
Boston city directories, 1818-1847; federal census schedules for Boston, 1840 and
1850, microfilm copy at the Federal Records Center, Waltham, Mass.: Records of
Marriages and Records of Deaths, Bureau of Vital Records, State House, Boston;
Boston City Valuation Books, 1827-1847, Boston Public Library. Before 1838,
property was listed at only 50 percent of its full value.
There were also forty-one women who joined the American Physiological
Society. But twenty-four of them were wives of male members, and several of
the rest were apparently their daughters. The Society was essentially a male organization.
8. Arthur Loesser, *Men, Women, and Pianos: A Social History* (New York,
1954), pp. 445-470; Rosamund E. M. Harding, *The Piano-Forte: Its History
Traced to the Great Exhibition of 1851* (Cambridge, [England], 1933); Daniel

Spillane, *History of the American Pianoforte: Its Technical Development, and the Trade* (New York, 1890); Daniel J. Boorstin, *The Americans: The National Experience* (New York, 1965), pp. 148-152.

9. Spillane, *The American Pianoforte*, pp. 165-167. In 1840 the Franklin Institute of Philadelphia awarded one of Brown's instruments the top honors among 21 entrants, commending its "superior" tone and calling its patented soft pedal "a very pleasing and effective innovation" (ibid., p. 166). A picture of one of Brown's instruments of the late 1840s—an extremely ornate square piano with elaborately curved legs and filigree decoration throughout—appears as part of an advertisement for his firm in *History and Sketches of Boston from 1650 to 1856* (Boston, 1851 [sic]), p. 99. Brown was still alive as late as 1890.

10. For a discussion of outmigration rates in Boston during the antebellum period, see Peter R. Knights, *The Plain People of Boston, 1830-1860: A Study in City Growth* (New York, 1971), pp. 103-118.

11. Russell Thacher Trall, "Biographical Sketch of Sylvester Graham," *Water-Cure Journal* 12 (1851): 110-111.

12. Ibid.; Northampton Town Papers Collection, 5.74, Forbes Library, Northampton, Mass. (I am indebted to Christopher Clark for bringing this document to my attention.) Graham owned five shares in the Connecticut Railroad Company and 204 shares in the Delaware and Hudson Canal Company. He was apparently exaggerating his financial troubles, if not his emotional ones: his net estate finally amounted to just over $20,000 (see Hampshire County, Mass., Registry of Probate, Box 62, no. 30).

13. For an account of William A. Alcott's sex books, see Sidney Ditzion, *Marriage, Morals and Sex in America* (New York, 1953), pp. 322-326.

14. A more complete explanation of phrenology, and an account of its American history, is John D. Davies, *Phrenology, Fad and Science: a 19th-century American Crusade* (New Haven, 1955). There is a detailed discussion of the early years of "scientific" phrenology in Boston, its American center, in three works by Anthony A. Walsh: "Johann Gaspar Spurzheim and the Rise and Fall of Scientific Phrenology in Boston, 1832-42" (Ph.D. diss., University of New Hampshire, 1974); "Phrenology and the Boston Medical Community in the 1830's," *Bulletin of the History of Medicine* 50 (1976): 261-273; and "The American Tour of Dr. Spurzheim," *Journal of the History of Medicine* 27 (1972): 187-205. An excellent discussion of the social implications of British phrenology is T. M. Parssinen, "Popular Science and Society: The Phrenology Movement in Early Victorian Britain," *Journal of Social History* (Fall 1974): 1-20.

15. Franz Gall, et al., *On the Functions of the Cerebellum* (Edinburgh, 1838).

16. Sylvester Graham, *Lectures on the Science of Human Life* 2 vols. (Boston, 1839), 2: 228-246. At another point, however, Graham reported the basic principles of phrenology without passing judgment on them (1: 359 ff).

17. F. J. V. Broussais, *Cours de Phrenologie* (Paris, 1836).

18. Orson S. Fowler, *Fowler on Temperance and Phrenology; or, The laws of life and the principles of the human constitution, as developed by the science*

of phrenology and physiology applied to total abstinence from all alcoholic and intoxicating drinks, 4th ed. (New York, 1845); Orson S. Fowler, *Matrimony; or, Phrenology and physiology applied to the selection of a suitable companion for life* (New York, 1841); Lorenzo Fowler, *The Principles of Phrenology and Physiology Applied to Man's Social Relations* (New York, 1842). For a discussion of the relationship between phrenology and Grahamism, see Davies, *Phrenology,* pp. 106-117; and on the relationship between Graham and the Fowler brothers, see Madeline B. Stern, *Heads and Headlines: The Phrenological Fowlers* (Norman, Okla., 1971), pp. 47-50.

19. Orson S. Fowler, *Physiology, Animal and Mental: applied to the preservation and restoratin of health of body, and power of mind* (New York, 1847), p. 67. Samuel R. Wells, another phrenologist and a business partner of Fowler, was a founder of both the American Vegetarian Society and the American Anti-Tobacco Society. (Davies, *Phrenology,* p. 109; Walker, "Health Reform," p. 203). Significantly, European phrenologists such as Spurzheim and Combe displayed no interest in what Fowler termed "physiology": the connection between the two was made, it seems, chiefly in America.

20. Orson S. Fowler, *Amativeness: or, Evils and remedies of excessive and perverted sexuality: including warning and advice to the married and single,* 12th ed. (New York, 1846); *Love and Parentage, Applied to the improvement of offspring,* 12th ed. (New York, 1846); and *Maternity, or The bearing and nursing of children* (New York, 1848). See also Orson S. Fowler's *Hereditary Descent* (New York, 1843). Fowler continued to write about sexual hygiene until the end of his life: see *Sexuality Restored* (Boston, 1870); *Private Lectures on Perfect Men Women and Children* (New York, 1880); and his major treatise on the subject, *Creative and Sexual Science* (New York, 1870)—a book of more than 1,000 pages. Other phrenologists who wrote similar works include Orson's brother, Lorenzo Fowler, *Marriage* (New York, 1847); Nelson Sizer, *Cupid's Eyes Opened* (New York, 1848); Samuel R. Wells, *Wedlock* (New York, 1869); John Cowen, *The Science of a New Life* (New York, 1869), *The Use of Tobacco vs. Purity, Chastity and Good Health* (New York, 1870), and *What All Married People Should Know* (Chicago, 1903); and Ray Vaughn Pierce, *The People's Common Sense Medical Advisor* (Buffalo, 1875). While Pierce was a physician rather than a practicing phrenologist, his book is filled with phrenological analysis.

21. Walker, "Health Reform," pp. 169-174. Joel Shew's first book, *Hydropathy; or, The water-cure* (New York, 1844), contained an appendix on "Animal and Vegetable Diet," filled with passages from Graham's *Lectures.* It is clear that Shew was a Grahamite before he discovered the water-cure (Shew, *Hydropathy,* pp. 275-304).

22. *Water-Cure Journal* 10 (1850): 15 (quoted in Walker, "Health Reform," p. 206); Walker, "Health Reform," pp. 212-213. Walker's work contains an excellent account of the genesis and progress of the hydropathic movement. See also Harry B. Weiss and Howard R. Kemble, *The Great American Water-Cure Craze: A history of hydropathy in the United States* (Trenton, N.J., 1967); and M. S. Legan, "Hydropathy in America: A 19th century Panacea," *Bulletin of the History of Medicine* 45 (1971): 267-280. For a perceptive as well as an entertaining discussion of the move-

ment's appeal to middle-class women of the 1840s see Kathryn Kish Sklar, "All Hail to Pure Cold Water," *American Heritage* 26 (1974): 64-69, 100-101.

23. See also Russell Thacher Trall, *Tobacco: Its history, nature and effects* (New York, 1854).

24. Walker, "Health Reform," pp. 176-180, 203-205.

25. *Water-Cure Journal* 18 (1854): 31; and 20 (1855): 66 (quoted in Walker, "Health Reform," pp. 231-234); Weiss and Kemble, *Water-Cure Craze,* p. 82.

26. See, for example, Russell Thacher Trall, *Home-Treatment for Sexual Abuses: A practical treatise* (New York, 1853), pp. iii-xii. There were several doctors who catered primarily or exclusively to individuals with sexual problems. Such physicians generally advertised their services by writing books and pamphlets on sexual subjects. Perhaps the three most prominent of these were Frederick Hollick (1818-1894), Edward Bliss Foote (1829-1906) and Ray Vaughn Pierce (1840- ?). See Frederick Hollick, *The Diseases of Women* (New York, 1847), *The Male Generative Organs* (New York, 1855?), *The Marriage Guide* (before 1860), and *The Origin of Life* (New York, 1845); Edward Bliss Foote, *Medical Common Sense; applied to . . . unhappiness in Marriage* (Boston, 1860), *Plain Home Talk* (New York, 1870), and *Physiological Marriage* (New York, 1876); Ray Vaughn Pierce, *The People's Common Sense Medical Advisor* (Buffalo, 1875).

27. These included Robert James Culverwell, *Guide to Health and Long Life* (New York, 1848), and *The Institutes of Marriage* (New York, 1846); Richard Dawson, *An Essay on Marriage* (London, 1845), and *An Essay on Spermatorrhoea* (London, 1846); Eli Peck Miller, *A Father's Advice* (New York, 1881), and *A Treatise on the Causes of Exhausted Vitality* (New York, 1867).

28. Gerald Carson, *Cornflake Crusade* (New York, 1957), pp. 61-67. The best study of "Our Home on the Hillside" is in Charles Bowden's unpublished study, "Broke Bodies: A Look at Some Nineteenth Century Notions about Health," Part One.

29. Ronald L. Numbers, *Prophetess of Health: A Study of Ellen G. White* (New York, 1974), pp. 38, 59-61, 81-94, 162-168. Numbers discusses White's *An Appeal to Mothers* (1864) on pp. 150-155.

30. Numbers, *Prophetess of Health,* pp. 94-104.

31. Ibid., pp. 111-117, 121-128.

32. The quotation can be found in John Harvey Kellogg, *The Itinerary of a Breakfast* (New York and London, 1926), p. 3.

33. Carson, *Cornflake Crusade,* pp. 71-146. The Post family of Battle Creek, like the Kelloggs, were Adventists. The "San" itself, as the Battle Creek Sanitarium was familiarly called by the thousands of debilitated men and women who visited it in the course of its sixty-year existence, was in a sense the final reincarnation of the Graham boardinghouse.

10. RADICALIZATION
OF THE GRAHAM SYSTEM

"God has made man free," proclaimed Thomas Low Nichols in 1853 in his book *Esoteric Anthropology*. "But instead of accepting this freedom . . . men have used [it] to destroy the freedom of each other." These were familiar words in Jacksonian America, and if Nichols had been referring to politics or religion, most of his compatriots could only have echoed the sentiment. But the freedom he intended was something else again: it was sexual freedom. And the institution he was attacking was associated not with tyrants or popes, but with the essence of republican virtue—monogamous marriage.

"Human passions," Nichols insisted, appropriating the rhetoric of American democracy and laissez-faire capitalism, "must have freedom for development, freedom of action, freedom of enjoyment." God has left these passions free, Nichols went on, so that they might "act by His attraction." But by inventing such artificial institutions as marriage, society has "bound and starved" them by "a system of restraints and repressions"; it has "loaded them with chains, and shut them up in prisons and in darkness." Marriage is nothing less than the tomb of passion, and in any case, "men and women find universally that their susceptibility to love is not burnt out by one honeymoon, or satisfied by one lover."[1]

Thomas Low Nichols was not the only American who was critical of marriage during the 1850s. Even in the previous decade a number of reformers had publicly theorized about the deficiencies of conventional sexual arrangements, and a few of them had gone so far as to implement alternatives they considered superior. Early in the 1840s Joseph Smith had startled his own Mormon followers as well as the rest of the nation by initiating a system of plural marriage. Shortly afterwards, John Humphrey Noyes had begun to practice what he called "complex marriage," first in his native Vermont community of Putney and later at Oneida in western New York.[2] During the same years, the widespread American popularity of the social theories of Charles Fourier caused some of his followers to identify marriage itself with the so-called isolated family (i.e., the nuclear household), which all Fourierites held in disfavor. (Most American Fourierites, however, including both Albert Brisbane and Horace Greeley, ignored and even denied the fact that Fourier himself wished to eliminate monogamous marriage.)

In 1849 Henry James, Sr., father of the novelist and an articulate disciple of both Fourier and Emanuel Swedenborg, published *Love in the Phalanstery*, the English translation of a work that depicted sexual arrangements under Fourierism.[3] But three years later, in reviewing a book that criticized marriage in terms considerably more extreme than his own, James denied that he had ever condemned marriage per se: all he really wished was to have the institution purified through a liberalization of the divorce laws. James's apparent retreat was challenged by Stephen Pearl Andrews, a follower of the philosophical anarchist Josiah Warren and a partisan of "individual sovereignty." In a three-way argument carried on by Andrews, James, and Horace Greeley in the pages of Greeley's newspaper, the *New York Tribune,* and later published in book form, Andrews argued that the only way to purify sexual relationships was by abolishing marriage itself. In 1851 Andrews had founded on Long Island the short-lived community of Modern Times, dedicated to the free and undirected expression of individual sovereignty, sexual and otherwise.[4]

But of all the people who wrote about sexual arrangements during this period, it was Thomas Low Nichols (1815-1884) who combined the most bitter condemnation of marriage with the most expansive celebration of human sexuality. Nichols's critique of marriage, in itself, was not very different from Andrews' critique, or even from that of James. (Indeed, together with his wife Mary, herself an articulate supporter of her husband's radical views, Nichols had been a member of the Modern Times community, and both husband and wife had been convinced Fourierites during the 1840s.) But his free-love program was rooted not only in the doctrines of "individual sovereignty" and communal existence, but also in an exaltation of sexual functions and relationships in themselves. To define adultery as a criminal act, Nichols contended in a phrase which pointed back to Stephen Pearl Andrews and beyond him into the previous century, was "a trespass on natural right." But Nichols did not stop with this kind of argument. He went on to insist, in language which suggested a wholly different world of discourse, that "what the law calls adultery, may be the highest and truest relation of which two persons are capable." In the same way, he argued that what the law calls fornication "may be the holiest action two human beings can engage in," and that the "real, essential nature of the act can be changed by no ceremony."[5]

Nichols considered sexuality to be the most rewarding of all human functions. "The influence of sex runs through the whole mental and moral character," he wrote. "The whole powers of body and soul are engaged in this function, which confers the greatest happiness upon the individual." At times Nichols sounded more as though he were writing in the middle of the twentieth century than in the middle of the nineteenth. He continually referred to the pleasure women took in sexual intercourse, and he maintained that their enjoyment could and should be as great as men's. Women are capable of deep and regular orgasms, and it is not unusual for them to attain "six or seven orgasms in rapid succession, each seeming to be more violent and ecstatic than the last." Nichols even acknowledged that women can take greater sexual satisfaction than men: there was "no doubt," he wrote, that "the pleasure of the female is longer continued, more frequently repeated, and more exquisite than that of the male."[6]

It is significant that the "violent" sensations and motions of orgasm suggested to Nichols exquisite pleasure and even ecstasy, and not the volcanic eruptions and pathological feelings they aroused in Sylvester Graham. In fact, the language with which Nichols described the effects of sexual excitement, intercourse, and orgasm could not be more different from Graham's words:

> The expressions of love antecedent to, and connected with its ultimation, are varied and beautiful, involving the whole being. Love gives light, and a trembling suffusion to the eye, a soft, tremulous tenderness to the voice, a sweet sadness to the demeanor, or a deep joyousness; a certain warmth and voluptuousness presides over the movements of the body; blushes come often to the cheeks, and the eyes are cast down with consciousness; the heart swells, and beats tumultuously . . . a new delight pervades the sense of feeling, which is more than any other the organ of this passion; every touch, even the hem of the garment, is a deep

pleasure; the hands clasp each other with a thrill of delight; the lips cling together in dewey kisses of inexpressible rapture; the bolder hands of man wander over the ravishing beauties of woman; he clasps her waist, he presses her soft bosom, and in a tumult of delirious ecstasy, each finds the central point of attraction and of pleasure, which increases until it is completed in the sexual orgasm—the most exquisite enjoyment of which the human senses are capable.[7]

But, for all that, it would be profoundly misleading to see the Nicholses as a kind of nineteenth-century anticipation of Masters and Johnson. What is even more striking about them than their ostensible modernity is the fact that their attitudes were, in the last analysis, rooted in the very spirit they appeared to reject. Their work had more in common with Sylvester Graham than with the epigones of the *Playboy* revolution. Their celebration of human sexuality was generally embedded in a wider context of fear and distrust, a context that suggests that Victorian sexual radicalism was just as Victorian as it was radical.

Take, for instance, Nichols's lyric description of sexual intercourse— the long passage just quoted. As it turns out, Nichols chose to follow this passage with a somber warning: precisely because sexual excitement is such an intense and consuming experience, it must be carefully "guarded against" under any circumstances "where it is desirable to avoid such excitement." A little later Nichols enumerated the kinds of dangerous circumstances he had in mind. His list included incomplete physical and intellectual maturity of either the man or the woman; the absence of mutual and deep love between them; the lack of financial resources sufficient to insure the "suitable nurture and education" of the child who might be conceived; a pelvis too small in the woman partner to permit easy delivery; and the presence in either partner of any hereditary defects or "distressing singularities of mind." (In this last category Nichols included "diseased amativeness"— a phrenological term denoting nymphomania and satyriasis. This meant, in effect, that wanting sex too much was itself sufficient reason for avoiding it!) Nichols indicated elsewhere that coitus should never be performed in the midst of illness, depression, or fatigue, or under "the influence of stimulants." It was to be altogether avoided, likewise—at the risk of doing irreparable damage to the unborn child or infant—during the entire course of pregnancy and lactation. (Since Nichols was in full agreement with

Orson Fowler and others that a child had to be nursed for two full years, it followed, altogether he never said so, that a couple would go without any sexual relations for the better part of three years each time they conceived a child.)[8]

Finally, Nichols added, even when all other conditions were ideal, sexual intercourse should be avoided if it had already taken place at a recent date, since overindulgence was as harmful as any other kind of abuse. Nichols stressed this point: "Amative excesses, even at a proper age, and under the proper circumstances, produce exhaustion, and so cause disease." (Like Graham, Nichols felt that sex was "exhausting," and that exhaustion produced disease.) He proposed, just as Graham had done, that intercourse be performed no more often than once every month. He warned married couples not to violate this rule even on their honeymoon. "Amative excess" at this time, he warned, might well mean that "permanent happiness is sacrificed to a few days of delirious and not very satifsying enjoyment."[9]

In short, if married couples followed Nichols's advice scrupulously through the course of their child-bearing years, they might have made love only as many times as the number of their children. Yet, strangely enough, this too was precisely what Nichols meant when he insisted that "human passions must have freedom for development, freedom of action, freedom of enjoyment."

Nichols laid down these strictures because he believed, as did Graham, that the very intensity of excitement that made sex the most powerful human experience also made it the most exhausting. "There is no passion so exhausting as amativeness." Nichols's debt to Graham extended even to his specific arguments and the terms in which he presented them. Along with Graham, for instance, Nichols emphasized that it was not the loss of semen that produced the exhaustion that resulted from sexual excess: it was the drainage of nervous energy. Too much sex, he maintained, renders "the nervous powers completely exhausted." Again, for all the phrenological terms and categories he was fond of using (the word "amative," for example), Nichols continued to employ Graham's distinction between the "animal" and the "organic" system. One example is this catalogue of the effects of sexual mismanagement (which is reminiscent of Graham's *Lecture on Chastity* in other ways as well):

> The abuse of amativeness [Nichols began] rapidly exhausts
> the nervous power. The generative function takes strength from
> the organic and animal powers. It fails, and all fail. The stomach

can not digest, for want of the nervous energy, spent in oft-repeated and fruitless orgasms. Nutrition can not be carried on in the capilary system. The waste matter . . . is retained to poison the fountain of life. The skin becomes dry and withered; the eye dull; the mind weak and disordered; all noble passions lose their force; the whole system is discord and disorder, and ready to become a prey to disease. Then comes epilepsy, or spinal disease, or dropsy, or some form of consumption . . . .[10]

Nichols devoted just as much effort as Graham to elaborating the physical and moral consequences of overindulgence. "The nervous exhaustion which it occasions," he wrote in one characteristic summary, "is the direct cause of most cases of dyspepsia, rheumatism, palsy, epilepsy, apoplexy, the nervous and uterine diseases of women, and, in fact, of two-thirds of all the diseases of mankind." Like overindulgence, masturbation too was a major cause of disease. It led to nocturnal emissions, palsy, insanity, heart attack, consumption, and epilepsy. "I have never seen a case of epilepsy that was not caused by amative excess, and generally by masturbation," wrote Nichols; and he made the same point about a variety of other ailments.[11]

Nichols advocated temperance and vegetarianism as ardently as he advocated free love. *Esoteric Anthropology* was filled with stern admonitions about the adverse effects of liquor, meat, tobacco, and other stimulants on sexual health—and on well-being in general. In addition to animal food and alcohol, Nichols noted that "salt, pepper, spices, and all stimulating substances, provoke to venery," and that "coffee stimulates the nervous system, and the stimulation is apt to take this [sexual] direction." In general, it was safe to say that "a full diet provokes to lust." Predictably enough, Nichols recommended "strict temperance, passional and dietetic," as the most effective remedy for virtually every symptom. He even advocated Graham's staple dietary principle—the regular use of "coarse bread" to soothe and regulate the system.[12]

Nichols's debt to Graham was no coincidence. By the time he published *Esoteric Anthropology* in 1853, both Nichols and his wife had been convinced and active Grahamites for almost twenty years. Nichols had first adopted Graham's doctrines in 1834, as a nineteen year-old freshman at Dartmouth College, when he heard a lecture delivered by Graham.[13] He left Dartmouth at the end of that academic year and tried to make his way into the world of New York City literary and political journalism. He published novels, stories, and a Democratic party campaign periodical, the *Young Hickory Banner.* But by the mid-1840s the direction of his commitment had shifted, and he became an energetic participant in a variety of movements for social and hygienic reform.

Nichols earned a medical degree at New York University in 1850. That same year he helped organize the American Vegetarian Society and became co-editor of its official publication, *The American Vegetarian and Health Journal.* His most active work during these years, however, was as a hydropathic theoretician and practitioner. Along with Joel Shew and Russell Thacher Trall, Nichols was the most prominent spokesman for the water-cure movement. (Inasmuch as both Shew and, especially, Trall wrote extensively on matters of sexual hygiene, it is possible to think of a work like *Esoteric Anthropology* as a hydropathic sex manual as well as an antimarriage tract.)

Together with his wife, whom he had married in 1847, Nichols helped to put out the *Water-Cure Journal and Herald of Reform* (published by Fowlers and Wells), and to run a variety of hydropathic establishments, first in New York and, after 1853, in Cincinnati. He also produced several volumes on the water-cure, including *An Introduction to the Water-Cure,* subtitled a "concise exposition of the human constitution, the conditions of health, etc." This book gave no hint that its author was about to challenge established sexual morality in the name of good health.

Mary Gove Nichols (1811-1902) arrived at her radical position with Grahamite credentials that were, if anything, even more solid than her husband's. In 1838, at the age of twenty-seven, she had opened a "Graham Boarding School" in Lynn, Massachusetts, and before the end of that year she was delivering "Lectures to Ladies on Anatomy and Physiology" at Boston. These lectures were essentially a briefer version of both Graham's *Lectures on the Science of Human Life* and his *Lecture on Chastity,* with special emphasis on the problems of women. Soon, Mary Gove—she had married a hat-maker named Hiram Gove in 1831, and would leave him a decade later—had become known as a kind of female equivalent to Sylvester Graham. This role was needed at the time, since Graham himself had gotten into serious difficulty in 1837 when he tried to speak about physiology to female audiences. An anonymous contributor to the *Graham Journal* had even wondered whether there might not be "some intelligent and tallented [sic] ladies" to do the job.

Mrs. Gove's lectures were successful, and she repeated them through New England, New York, and Pennsylvania during 1839. They were summarized (with the sexual material omitted) in the *Graham Journal,* and published in book form in 1842.[14]

At the beginning of 1840, by this time permanently separated from her husband, she founded her own periodical, the *Health Journal and Advocate of Physiological Reform,* published at Worcester and Boston. Filled with praise of Graham's work and with extensive quotations from his *Lectures on the Science of Human Life* at the very time when his personal popularity was rapidly waning, the magazine failed within a year. Continuing to lecture, Mary Gove discovered the water-cure movement soon after it emerged on the American scene in 1844. She moved to New York City, where she studied hydropathic technique for a short time with Joel Shew, and in 1845 she opened her own water-cure establishment there on Tenth Street.

During these years Mrs. Gove involved herself in the New York literary and intellectual world. She became friendly with Edgar Allen Poe, and published several stories in *Godey's Lady's Book* as well as three novels. At the same time she was on the editorial board of the *Phalanx,* a journal of Fourierite theory. In 1847 she met Thomas Low Nichols and married him shortly after obtaining a divorce from her first husband. After their marriage, in addition to the projects they pursued jointly, Mary Gove Nichols continued to write under her own name on both hygienic and literary topics. When Nichols published *Marriage* in 1854, the passages in that book that most bitterly attacked conventional morality were those contained in a section written by his wife.

Figures such as Thomas Low Nichols and Mary Gove Nichols present a real problem. On the same page they were capable of rhapsodizing about sexual life and castigating it, of condemning marriage in the name of sexual freedom and condemning the exercise of sexual freedom in the name of health. What makes this paradox significant as well as interesting is the fact that it was more than the personal idiosyncracy of a single individual, or a single couple. It constituted, in fact, the central tension of mid-nineteenth century American sexual radicalism. It is impossible to locate a single figure who attacked marriage during this period (and difficult to find many figures who defended it) whose sexual doctrines were free of this tension. Stephen Pearl Andrews's were not, nor were

Joseph Smith's.[15] But the tension appeared in what was perhaps its most striking form in the system instituted by John Humphrey Noyes among his followers at Putney and Oneida.

On the one hand, Noyes celebrated sexual desire—he, too, called it "amativeness"—as "the first and noblest of the social affections," and his system of "complex marriage" permitted and even encouraged any consenting man and woman to engage in sexual relations with each other at any time. But on the other hand, Noyes qualified this arrangement by establishing another principle, which he called "male continence." The male partner in a sexual act was not permitted to achieve, or even approach, an orgasm. Instead, upon entering the woman he was to remain motionless until his erection had subsided naturally, minutes or hours later.[16] Noyes justified this practice on the grounds that sexual intercourse actually consisted of two physiologically distinct acts—the "amative" and the "propagative." The "propagative" act (that is, male orgasm), was merely sensual, and it was potentially dangerous to health. By eliminating it from coitus, it became possible to "stop the drain of life on the part of man." In any case, orgasm was unnecessary since the "amative" part of sexual intercourse (that is, the presence of the penis in the vagina) was a "distinct and independent act" which amounted to a "simple union of persons." Noyes thought of true sexual intercourse as "a quiet affair, like conversation."[17]

Just as much as Sylvester Graham, then, despite their difference in style, John Humphrey Noyes wished to desensualize sex. It is significant that this attempted desensualization took place on both extremes of the ideological spectrum—and that it was intended to apply to men as well as to women. The distrust of sexuality and sexual excitement which was publicly articulated by Sylvester Graham came to dominate the culture of mid-nineteenth century America so deeply that it pervaded the sensibility of even the most unconventional sexual theorists of the age.

In fact, Grahamite attitudes not only formed the thinking of sexual radicals; it actually provided much of the impetus that led them to reject conventional marriage in the first place. Graham himself was able to devise, after all, only the most tenuous and unsatisfactory justification of marriage. All it amounted to, really, was the assurance that while all sex was inherently harmful, marital sex was less harmful than other kinds— less harmful to the degree that it was less enjoyable. For all Graham's protestations, this was scarcely the most forceful way to clinch the point that monogamous marriage was "founded in the constitutional nature of things." But even though the argument was unconvincing as an apology for marriage, Graham nevertheless staked his entire defense of the institution on it. Time and again he insisted that while marriage might be enjoined by both biblical and civil law, it was ultimately founded—like the Bible and the civil order themselves—"on the physiological principles established in the constitutional nature of man."

But in his desire to refute such infidel antimarriage theorists as Robert Dale Owen on their own naturalistic terms, Graham overextended himself, and he unwittingly managed to enhance the force of their own conclusions. To condemn marriage with Graham's own logic, after all, it was necessary only to carry his argument a single step further than he carried it himself: to deny either that marital sex really *was* ordinarily less exciting than masturbation, adultery, or fornication, or that it occurred less frequently. (Indeed, Graham himself had insisted that marital excess was increasing dramatically in the nineteenth century.) As soon as this step was taken, marriage stood condemned on the very grounds by which Graham had attempted to preserve it.

It was just this kind of reasoning that helped bring the Nicholses to the point where, by the early 1850s, they believed marriage to be incompatible with a healthy and moral society. As they saw it, marriage permitted and even encouraged the most brutal and debilitating sexual abuses, especially toward women. It led, for instance, to the performance of sexual acts during the period of pregnancy and lactation—a practice which often did lasting harm to the health of the unborn child or nursing infant. "Among the veriest savages," Nichols wrote—along with Graham and other Jacksonian reformers, he believed that primitive cultures were generally superior to modern society in such matters—"a woman is considered sacred from the demands of sexual passion from the beginning of her pregnancy until her babe is weaned." In bleak constrast, "our monogamic marriage knows no such sanctity of the maternal function, and women are compelled to bear what no animal even, in its natural state, ever submits to."[18]

But the sexual degradation imposed by marriage extended beyond periods of pregnancy and lactation. Marriage amounted to little more than sexual slavery—and ordinarily (though not always) it was the wife who was the slave. No matter how little a woman might wish to respond to the "morbid passions" of her husband, even if they struck her as utterly

"loathsome," she was obliged to "submit to his embraces."[19] Where
sex was all morbid lust on the one hand, and all loathing on the other,
the result was only too predictable: debilitation and disease. "The whole
train of what are called female diseases," suggested Nichols, "are mainly
caused by the legalized and sanctified brutalities of civilized marriage."[20]
To this claim his wife added a graphic demonstration:

> In the Medical College, at Albany, there is an exposition of in-
> dissoluble marriage, which should be studied by all those who
> begin to see that a legalized union may be a most impure, unholy,
> and, consequently, unhealthy thing. . . . In glass vases, ranged in
> a large cabinet in this medical museum, are uterine tumors, weigh-
> ing from half a pound to twenty-four pounds. A viscus that in its
> ordinary state weighs a few ounces, is brought, by the disease
> caused by amative excess—in other words, licentiousness and im-
> purity—to weigh more than twenty pounds.

"Be it remembered," Mrs. Nichols concluded, "these monstrosities were
produced in lawful and indissoluble wedlock."[21]

The bad consequences of marriage were psychological as well as
physical. Husbands and wives, aware that their connection was indissoluble,
often lost all concern with appearing attractive or acting pleasant to each
other. In this way marriage easily led to "such vices as uncleanliness,
slovenliness, uncouth actions, and degrading habits, as the use of foul
language, ardent spirits, or tobacco." In fact, Nichols claimed, "more
men and women have been made drunkards by the exhaustion, monotony
and disgust of a false indissoluble marriage, than by all other causes combined." (This was surely a cause of drinking Sylvester Graham had never
investigated.) Moreover, by virtually forcing couples to engage in sexual
intercourse under such circumstances, marriage "breeds salacity and ob-
scenity," and it is therefore ultimately responsible for the prevalence of
"masturbation, prostitution, and general licentiousness."[22]

Hostility, drunkenness, and infidelity were the inevitable consequences
of a legal relationship that could be severed by death alone. The Nicholses
condemned marriage in the very name of conventional virtue and morality.
But what about the system of free love with which they proposed to replace it? Would such a system not lead to promiscuity and excess at
least as degrading as that within marriage itself? Not in the least, Mary

Gove Nichols responded: "Do you think that women are so sensual that they would rush into promiscuous intercourse, when now, more than nine-tenths deprecate sexual union as a great evil, and do not wish to have children?"[23]

For Mary Gove Nichols, "free love" effectively meant the freedom *not* to love—or, more specifically, not to *make* love.[24] It meant the freedom to refuse to submit to the sexual requirements of marriage, requirements enforceable by law. This was the essence of her radicalism. And in it she was supported by her husband, who whole-heartedly agreed with her claim that "sensuality would be much lessened by freedom." Thomas Low Nichols, too, regarded free love, at least for women, as "the negative right of refusing to live with those whom they do not love." Even for men, he insisted that "freedom would result in a more healthful moderation" of sexual activity than was possible under the system of monogamous marriage. This moderation would come about, he suggested, through an entirely natural process. "The greater the repression of any natural desire, the more inordinate becomes any permitted gratification." For this reason, "the amative propensity attains a morbid activity in the constraints and repressions of civilization." It was just such morbid activity that sexual freedom would relieve. "Freedom, let us repeat the thousandth time, is not licentiousness, but is the only safeguard of purity and virtue."[25]

As it happened, freedom was not an adequate safeguard of purity and virtue. In 1856 Dr. and Mrs. Nichols founded an experimental community at Yellow Springs, Ohio, at which they determined to put their system to the test. Against the bitter objections of Horace Mann, president of newly-founded Antioch College, they proclaimed full sexual liberty for the small band of followers—most of them students at their earlier hydropathic institutes—who accompanied them to "Memnonia," as they named their community. But within three months the couple had decided that the members of the community were not yet spiritually prepared for the life of freedom—the corrupt influence of civilized culture had touched too deep—and they announced the "temporary" imposition for the entire membership of total and unqualified celibacy.

This new celibate regimen was still in effect when Mary Gove Nichols received a "message" from the ghost of St. Ignatius Loyola—the couple were both convinced spiritualists—ordering her to investigate the doctrines of the Roman Catholic Church. She did so over a period of several months, and early in 1857, along with her husband and several of their followers, she formally became a member of the Church. "Memnonia" was immediately disbanded, and the Nicholses spent the next few years lecturing on diet and health to Roman Catholic audiences in different parts of the country.[26] They moved to England shortly after the outbreak of the Civil War.

In England, their former radicalism unsuspected, they continued their careers in dietary and sexual hygiene. Nichols edited the *Herald of Health* (published in London) from 1875 to 1886, and for a while he ran a "health depot" in that city, selling Graham flour and other health foods. As if to suggest that their reformation was complete, the Nicholses published in 1873 a new edition of *Esoteric Anthropology* which contained not the slightest hint of their earlier condemnation of marriage or their espousal of free love. So thoroughly did Dr. and Mrs. Nichols cover their intellectual tracks—that one modern historian, evidently unaware of their American careers and basing his judgment primarily on the later edition of *Esoteric Anthropology,* has considered them perfect representatives of "the most extreme sort of sexuality respectability" to be found in mid-Victorian England.[27] In a certain sense, his judgment applies with equal force to their earlier, radical phase.

NOTES

1. Thomas Low Nichols, *Esoteric Anthropology: A comprehensive and confidential treatise on the structure, functions, passional attractions and perversions, true and false physical and social conditions, and the most intimate relations of men and women* (New York, 1853); 2nd ed. (New York, 1855), p. 256. Thomas Low Nichols and Mary Gove Nichols, *Marriage: Its history, character, and results* (Cincinnati, 1854), p. 128.

2. For full accounts of theory and practice in both Mormon polygamy and Oneidan complex marriage, see Raymond Lee Muncy, *Sex and Marriage in Utopian Communities* (Bloomington, Ind., 1973), chapters 9-12.

3. Victor Hennequin, *Les amours au phalanstere* (Paris, 1847); and *Love in the Phalanstery* (New York, 1849). Henry James, Sr.'s translation was anonymous.

4. Stephen Pearl Andrews, *Love, Marriage and Divorce, and the Sovereignty of the Individual* (New York, 1853). The book that led to this three-way debate after James had reviewed it was written by a New York physician who, like James himself, was both a Fourierite and a Swedenborgian: M. Edgeworth Lazarus, *Love vs. Marriage* (New York, 1852). Lazarus also was the author of a book on *Involuntary Seminal Losses* (New York, 1852), as well as one on *Passional Hygiene and Natural Medicine* (New York, 1852). Like James, Lazarus had undoubtedly read Swedenborg's

Conjugial Love, which had been published in New York in 1846 as *Conjugal Love and Its Chaste Delights.* A slightly later attack on marriage from a similar position is Austin Kent, *Free-Love: or, A philosophical demonstration of the non-exclusive feature of connubial love* (Hopkinton, N.Y., 1857). See also any number of books written by the spiritualists of this period, many of whom had begun as Fourierites and/or Swedenborgians and incorporated antimarriage theory into their spiritualism. For a good account of the James-Greeley-Andrews debate, of Lazarus's *Love vs. Marriage,* and of the relationship of Fourierism, Swedenborgianism, and spiritualism to free-love doctrines, see Sidney Ditzion, *Marriage, Morals and Sex in America* (New York, 1953), pp. 137-157. See also Grace Kinkle Adams and Edward Hutter, *The Mad Forties* (New York, 1942), pp. 177-260. The Modern Times experiment is discussed in Muncy, *Sex and Marriage,* pp. 204-206, and Madeline B. Stern, *The Pantarch: A Biography of Stephen Pearl Andrews* (Austin, Texas, 1968), pp. 73-86.

5. Nichols and Nichols, *Marriage,* pp. 184-185.

6. Nichols, *Esoteric Anthropology,* pp. 53, 85, 153, 200, 204; see also Nichols and Nichols, *Marriage,* pp. 284-285.

7. Nichols, *Esoteric Anthropology,* pp. 152-153.

8. Ibid., pp. 150, 153, 234-238, 347-348, 437-438. In his concern for the effects of parental sexual activity on offspring, Nichols is typical of most sexual writers of the age, including Graham. See Orson S. Fowler, *Maternity, or the Bearing and Nursing of Children* (New York, 1848), and *Love and Parentage Applied to the Improvement of Offspring,* 12th ed. (New York, 1846); Alexander Walker, *Intermarriage: or, The mode in which . . . beauty, health and intellect result from certain unions, and deformity, disease, and insanity from others* (New York, 1839); Hester Pendleton, *The Parents' Guide for the Transmission of Desired Qualities to Offspring* (New York, 1848), and *Husband and Wife; or, The science of human development through inherited tendencies* (New York, 1863); and [?] Porter, *Book of Men, Women and Babies* (New York, 1855). Both of Mrs. Pendleton's books were published by Fowlers and Wells, the earlier one as part of the "Water-Cure Library."

It should also be noted that physiological versions of the "sins-of-the-fathers" principle were often advanced by medical theorists as justifications for female subordination. Female education, these doctors argued, threatened to create a class of potential wives whose reproductive organs had been left underdeveloped because of the diversion of needed vital energy to their brains. With logic similar to that Graham applied to young people in general, they added the probability that an overeducated (and thus mentally overexcitable) woman would suffer from excess of sexual desire. Her children would therefore be twice as likely to contract debilitating ailments in the womb, and render her own education doubly counterproductive. For examples of this type of thinking and estimates of its importance as a rationalization for Victorian sex-role stereotypes, see Graham Barker-Benfield, *Horrors of the Half-Known Life* (New York, 1976), pp. 54-55; Charles Rosenberg and Carroll Smith-Rosenberg, "The Female Animal: Medical and Biological Views of Woman and Her Role in 19th Century America," *Journal of American History* 60 (1973): 332-356; and John S. Haller, Jr. and Robin M. Haller, *The Physician and Sexuality in Victorian America* (Urbana, Ill., 1974), pp. 131-137.

9. Nichols, *Esoteric Anthropology*, pp. 149, 234, 270. To be sure, Nichols allows once a week as the *absolute* maximum frequency, assuming that all other indications are positive (p. 200).

10. Ibid., pp. 268-269, 398-399.

11. Ibid., pp. 269, 355, 357-358, 373, 392-393, 418-419.

12. Ibid., pp. 199, 248-249, 357-361.

13. This biographical sketch of Dr. Nichols, along with the following sketch of Mary Gove Nichols, is taken from Bertha-Monica Stearns, "Two Forgotten New England Reformers," *New England Quarterly* 6(1933): 59-84; Adams and Hutter, *The Mad Forties* (this book is a "non-fiction novel" organized around the career of Mrs. Nichols—a career associated with virtually every reform movement that flourished between 1830 and 1860); and Walker, "Health Reform," pp. 148-160, 217-220 (which contains the most exhaustive account of Mrs. Nichols's early career). See also Pamela Ridder, "Mary Gove Nichols and Health Reform, 1838-1855" (B.A. thesis, Harvard University, 1977).

14. Mary S. Gove, *Lectures to Ladies on Anatomy and Physiology* (Boston, 1842); *Graham Journal* 2 (1838): 128, 248, 272; 3 (1839), 20, 37.

15. See, for instance, Andrews, *Love, Marriage and Divorce*, pp. 16-19; and, on the Mormons, see Muncy, *Sex and Marriage*, pp. 134, 158.

16. This practice was publicized at a later date as *karezza;* it is a form of what is technically known as *coitus reservatus*. (The latter denotes the avoidance only of the orgasm, and not necessarily of intravaginal movement.) In no case should it be confused, as Noyes's enemies often appeared to confuse it, with *coitus interruptus,* in which the male does achieve an orgasm but withdraws his penis immediately before it comes on. *Coitus interruptus* is almost invariably employed as a means of contradeption, and Noyes made it plain that "male continence" was not intended primarily for this purpose. See John Humphrey Noyes, "Male Continence" (Oneida, 1872), pp. 2-8. For an account of previous and subsequent uses of the technique, see Norman Himes, *A Medical History of Contraception* (Baltimore, 1936), pp. 127, 132, 269-271. See also Alice B. Stockham, *Karezza* (Chicago, 1896).

17. Noyes, "Male Continence," pp. 15-17. This section was originally published in 1848 as part of a short book titled *The Bible Argument*. Noyes also wrote an essay about Graham's theory of sexual excitement, published in one of his many short-lived early periodicals, *The Spiritual Moralist* (May 1842). Recent accounts of Noyes's sexual theories include Muncy, *Sex and Marriage,* pp. 182-183; and, especially, Robert David Thomas, *The Man Who Would Be Perfect: John Humphrey Noyes and the Utopian Impulse* (Philadelphia, 1977), chapter 5. (Thomas discusses the Noyes-Graham relationship on pp. 61-63.)

18. Nichols and Nichols, *Marriage,* pp. 185-186.

19. Ibid., pp. 75-85.

20. Ibid., p. 93.

21. Ibid., p. 207. There were other kinds of monstrosities "produced in lawful and indissoluble wedlock," too, as Mrs. Nichols pointed out.

> The hereditary evils to children born in a sensual and unloving marriage are everywhere visible. They are written in every lineament of the Present,—

sensuality, sickness, suffering, weakness, imbecility, or outrageous crime. I speak what I know, and testify what I have seen in a long and varied medical practice, when I assert that masturbation in children, and every evil of sensuality, spring from the polluted hotbed of a sensual and unloving marriage, where woman is subjected to a destroying sensualism during pregnancy and lactation (p. 223).

22. Ibid., pp. 129, 359; see also pp. 202, 228; and Nichols, *Esoteric Anthropology*, p. 212.

23. Nichols and Nichols, *Marriage*, p. 222.

24. It is important to observe here that, inasmuch as Mrs. Nichols saw husbands as the usual initiators of "loathsome embraces," there was a strong feminist tone to her formulations. In this regard the motivation behind Mrs. Nichols's sexual radicalism and the social conservatism of the female "moral reformers" of the Jacksonian period appear quite similar. As Carroll Smith-Rosenberg has pointed out, the latter group's theory of the causes of prostitution put primary emphasis on male "animality," and its tactics for eradicating the vice put special stress on intimidating male customers. See Carroll Smith-Rosenberg, "Beauty, the Beast, and the Militant Woman: A Case Study in Sex Roles and Social Stress in America," *American Quarterly* 23 (1971): 562-584. Even Orson S. Fowler, the phrenologist and author, wrote that "man should never obtrude on woman, but simply hold himself in readiness, subject to those invitations which woman knows full well how to give. . . . She, then, is that final umpire by which every husband should never fail to abide. . . ." Fowler, *Love and Parentage*, p. 134.

25. Nichols and Nichols, *Marriage*, pp. 345, 365-366.

26. Bertha-Monica Stearns, "Memnonia: The Launching of a Utopia," *New England Quarterly* 15 (1942): 280-295; Philip Gleason, "From Free-Love to Catholicism: Dr. and Mrs. Thomas L. Nichols at Yellow Springs," *Ohio Historical Quarterly* 70 (1961): 283-307.

27. Peter Cominos, "Late-Victorian Sexual Respectability and the Social System," *International Review of Social History*, 8 (1963): 18-48, 216-250; quoted phrase on p. 21. Representative later titles by the Nicholses include *Human Physiology, The basis of sanitary and social science* (London, 1872), *How to Cook* (London, 1872), *Dyspepsia* (n.p., 1884), and *Health* (London, 1884).

BIBLIOGRAPHY

SEXUAL HYGIENE LITERATURE IN AMERICA, 1830-1880

The following bibliography is both more and less than a list of the sources used in writing this book. It is a comprehensive inventory, though by no means a complete one, of the literature that sustained and conventionalized the feelings about human sexuality first publicly articulated by Sylvester Graham. Included are all the writings I have discovered, both popular and scientific, that deal directly with sexual hygiene and its physiological basis together with some other items on related subjects by important writers, about sexuality. The list is restricted to works published (though not necessarily written) in America between 1830 and 1880. It does not include works dealing primarily with the treatment of venereal disease. For works published before 1830, see Section 2 of the Bibliography.

Alcott, William A. *The Laws of Health*. Boston, 1857.
——. *Moral Philosophy of Courtship and Marriage*. Boston and Cleveland, 1857.
——. *The Physiology of Marriage*. Boston, 1856.
——. *Tea and Coffee*. Boston, 1839.
——. *The Use of Tobacco, Its physical, intellectual and moral effects on the human system*. New York, 1836.
——. *Vegetable Diet: As sanctioned by medical men, and by experience in all ages*. Boston, 1838.
——. *The Young Man's Guide*. Boston, 1834.
——. *The Young Woman's Book of Health*. Boston, 1850.
Andrews, Stephen Pearl. *Love, Marriage and Divorce, and the Sovereignty*

of the Individual; A discussion by Henry James, Horace Greeley, and S. P. Andrews, including the final replies of Mr. Andrews, rejected by the Tribune. New York, 1853.

——. "An Oration Delivered on the Fourth of July 1835, Before the East Feliciana Temperance Society at the Union Church, near Clinton, Louisiana."

Ayres, H. P. "Self-Pollution in Children," *Transactions of the Indiana Medical Society* (Indianapolis), 21 (1871): 161-179.

Baker, E. L. "A Few Cases Illustrative of the Ill Effects of Onanism," *Southern Medical and Surgical Journal* (Augusta), 2 (1846): 335-338.

Barr, R. N. "Spermatorrhoea," *Ohio Medical and Surgical Journal* (Columbus), 7 (1854-1855): 173-181.

Bartholomew, Roberts. "On the Pathology and Treatment of Spermatorrhoea," *Cincinnati Journal of Medicine* 1 (1866): 21, 78, 225, 288.

——. *On Spermatorrhoea.* New York, 1866.

Bauer, L. "Dementia Brought on by Excessive Self-Abuse; Cure by Infibulation," *St. Louis Clinical Record* 4 (1878): 271-273.

Beard, George Miller. *American Nervousness, Its Causes and Consequences.* New York, 1881.

——. *Eating and Drinking; A popular manual of food and diet in health and disease.* New York, 1871.

——. *Sexual Neurasthenia. Its hygiene, causes, symptoms, and treatment, with a chapter on diet for the nervous.* New York, 1884.

——. *Stimulants and Narcotics; Medically, philosophically, and morally considered.* New York, 1871.

——. *The Symptoms of Sexual Exhaustion.* Baltimore, 1880.

Bemise, Samuel Merrifield. "Epilepsy; Seminal Losses; Self-Pollution During Sleep," *New Orleans Journal of Medicine* 22 (1869), 729-731.

Bergeret, Louis Francois Etienne. *The Preventive Obstacle; or, Conjugal Onanism. The dangers and inconveniences to the individual, to the family, and to society, of frauds in the accomplishment of the generative functions.* New York, 1870.

Bigelow, Henry Jacob. "Castration as a Means of Cure for Satyriasis," *Boston Medical and Surgical Journal* 61 (1859-1860): 165.

Bolles, J. N. *Solitary Vice Considered.* New York, 1831 or 1832.

Bond, H. "Excessive Venery; Softening of the Brain," *Boston Medical and Surgical Journal* 36 (1847): 41.

Bond, Henry. "Note on the post mortem examination of a female who committed suicide almost immediately after coitus," *American Journal of Medical Science* (Philadelphia), 13 (1833): 403.

Calhoun, George R. *Report of the Consulting Surgeon on Spermatorrhoea, or seminal weakness, impotence, the vice of onanism, masturbation, or self-abuse, and other diseases of the sexual organs.* Philadelphia, 1858.

Chipley, William S. *A warning to fathers, teachers, and young men, in relation to a fruitful cause of insanity and other serious disorders of youth.* Louisville, Ky., 1861.

Cleaveland, Charles Hurley, "The Prevalence of Masturbation, and its Influence on Health," *New Hampshire Journal of Medicine* (Concord), 2 (1851-1852): 29-36.

Cooke, Nicholas Francis. *Satan in Society. By a Physician.* Cincinnati and New York, 1872.

Cornell, William Mason. *The Beacon; or, A warning to young and old. How body and mind are destroyed by evil habits, resulting in epilepsy, consumption, idiocy, and insanity.* Philadelphia, 1865.

Cowan, John. *The Science of a New Life.* New York, 1869.

——. *The Use of Tobacco vs. Purity, Chastity and Sound Health.* New York, 1870.

——. *What to Eat and How to Cook It.* New York, 1870.

Culverwell, Robert James. *Guide to Health and Long Life: Or, What to eat, drink, and avoid; What Exercise to Take, How to Control and Regulate the Passions and Appetites. . . .* New York, 1848.

——. *Hydropathy, Or the Cold Water Cure . . . .* London, 1842.

——. *Professional Records. The Institutes of Marriage, Its Intent, Obligations, and Physical and Constitutional Disqualifications, Anatomically, Physiologically, and Medically Considered. . . .* New York, 1846.

Davis, Andrew Jackson. *The Great Harmonia, Vol. IV, The Reformer: Concerning Physiological Vices and Virtues, and the Seven Phases of Marriage.* New York, 1855.

Deslandes, Leopold. *Manhood; The Causes of its Premature Decline. . . ; Addressed to Those Suffering from . . . Excessive Indulgence, Solitary Habits, etc.* Boston, 1843.

Dixon, Edward H., M.D. *The Organic Law of the Sexes. Positive and Negative Electricity, and the Abnormal Conditions that Impair Virility.* New York, 1861.

Donaldson, Francis. "Remarks on Onanism," *Virginia Medical Journal* (Richmond), 8 (1857): 390-399.

Dubois, Jean, M.D. *The Secret Habits of the Female Sex; Letters Addressed to a Mother of Girls on the Evils of Solitude and its Seductive Temptations to Young Girls, the Premature Victims of a Pernicious Passion. . . . Entailing Disease and Death.* N.P., 1848.

Duffey, Eliza Bisbee. *The Relations of the Sexes.* New York, 1876.

——. *What Women Should Know.* New York, pre-1876.

Earl, William. *Consumption: Its Causes, Nature, and Rational Treatment.* New York, 1878.

——. *The New Illustrated Silent Friend: Being a Complete Guide to Health, Marriage, and Happiness.* New York, 1858.

Everett, George H., M.D. and Susan Everett, M.D. *Health Fragments or, Steps Toward a True Life. Embracing Health, Digestion, Disease, and the Science of the Reproductive Organs.* New York, 1874.

Facts, and important information, from distinguished physicians and other sources, showing the awful effects of masturbation on young men. Boston, 1843.

Fleming, L.D. *Self-Pollution, The Cause of Youthful Decay; Showing the Dangers and Remedy of Venereal Exercise.* New York, 1846.

Foote, Edward Bliss. *Medical Common Sense; Applied to the Causes, Prevention and Cure of Chronic Diseases and Unhappiness in Marriage.* Boston, 1860.

——. *Physiological Marriage, An Essay Designed to Set People Thinking.* New York, 1876.

——. *Plain Home Talk About the Human System—The Habits of Men and Women; The Causes and Prevention of Disease; Our Sexual Relations and Social Natures . . . The Natural Relation of Men and Women to Each Other, Society, Love, Parentage (etc.).* New York, 1870.

Forwood, William Stump. "Onanism," *Medical and Surgical Reporter* (Philadelphia), 38 (1878): 44.

Fowler, Lorenzo. *Marriage: Its History and Ceremonies, with a Phrenological and Physiological Exposition of the Functions and Qualifications for Happy Marriages.* New York, 1847.

Fowler, Orson S. *Amativeness; or Evils and Remedies of Excessive and Perverted Sexuality.* 12th ed. New York, 1846.

——. *Hereditary Descent: Its Laws and Facts Applied to Human Improvement.* New York, 1847.

——. *Love and Parentage, Applied to the Improvement of Offspring, Including Important Directions and Suggestions to Lovers and the Mar-*

ried Concerning the Strongest Ties and the Most Momentous Relations of Life. New York, 1843.

——. *Maternity: or the Bearing and Nursing of Children. Including Female Education and Beauty.* New York, 1848.

——. *Matrimony: Or Phrenology and Physiology Applied to the Selection of a Suitable Companion for Life.* New York, 1841.

——. *O. S. Fowler on Temperance Founded on Phrenology and Physiology; Or, the Laws of Life and the Principles of the Human Constitution, as Developed by the Science of Phrenology and Physiology, Applied to Total Abstinence from all Alcoholic and Intoxicating Drinks.* Philadelphia, 1841.

——. *Physiology, Animal and Mental: Applied to the Preservation and Restoration of Health of Body, and Power of Mind.* New York, 1847.

——. *Practical Phrenology: Giving a Concise Elementary View of Phrenology; Presenting Some New and Important Remarks Upon the Temperaments; and Describing the Primary Mental Powers in Seven Different Degrees of Development; The Mental Phenomena Produced by their Combined Action; and the Location of the Organs, Amply Illustrated by Cuts. Also the Phrenological Developments, Together with the Character and Talents, of* [name to be filled in] *on* [date to be filled in]. New York, 1855.

——. *Private Lectures on Perfect Men, Women, and Children, in Happy Families; Including Gender, Love, Mating, Married Life and Reproduction, or Paternity, Maternity, Infancy and Puberty; Together with Male Vigor and Female Health Restored and their Ailments Self-cured.* New York, 1880.

——. *Sexuality Restored and Warning and Advice to Youth Against Perverted Amativeness; Including its Prevention and Remedies, as Taught by Phrenology and Physiology.* Boston, 1870.

——. *Creative and Sexual Science.* New York, 1870.

Gardner, Augustus Kinsley. *Conjugal Sins Against the Laws of Life and Health and Their Effects upon the Father, Mother, and Child.* New York, 1870.

Garwood, A. "A Case of Onanism in a Boy Seven Years Old," *Northwestern Medical and Surgical Journal* (Chicago), 11 (1854): 59-61.

Graham, Sylvester. *The Aesculapian Tablets of the Nineteenth Century.* Providence, 1834.

——. *Health from Diet and Exercise.* New York, n.d.

——. *A Lecture to Young Men, on Chastity, intended also for the serious consideration of parents and guardians.* Providence, 1834.

——. *A Lecture on Epidemic Diseases Generally, and Particularly the Spasmodic Cholera, delivered in . . . New York, March, 1832.* New York, 1833.

——. *Lectures on the Science of Human Life.* 2 vols. Boston, 1839.

——. "Thy Kingdom Come; A discourse on the importance of infant and Sunday Schools, delivered at Philadelphia, December 13, 1829." Philadelphia, 1831.

——. *A Treatise on Bread, and Bread-Making.* Boston, 1837.

Gregory, Samuel. *Facts and important information for young women, on the self-indulgence of the sexual appetite, its destructive effects on health, exciting causes, prevention, and cure.* 11th ed. Boston, 1857.

Haines, J. "Case of Onanism in a Child Five Years Old," *Western Medical-Chirurgical Journal* (Keokuk), 1 (1850): 330-333.

Hall, Alfred G. *Womanhood: Causes of its premature decline, respectfully illustrated. Being a review of the changes and derangements of the female constitution, a safe and faithful guide to mothers, during gestation, before and after confinement, with medical advice of the most salutary and important nature, to all females. . . .* 2nd ed. Rochester, 1845.

Hayes, Albert H. *A Medical Treatise on Nervous Affections.* Boston, 1870.

——. *The Science of Life; or Self-Preservation. A medical treatise on nervous and physical disability, spermatorrhoea, impotence, and sterility, with practical observations on the treatment of diseases of the generative organs.* Boston, 1868.

Henry, George W. *The Marriage of the Lamb, or Wedlock and Padlock, Temporal and Spiritual.* Oneida, 1856.

Hitchcock, Alfred. "Insanity and Death from Masturbation," *Boston Medical and Surgical Journal,* 26 (1842): 283-286.

——. "Insanity Produced by Masturbation," *Boston Medical and Surgical Journal,* 12 (1835): 105-111.

Holbrook, Martin Luther. *Marriage and Parentage and the Sanitary and Physiological Laws for the Production of Children of Finer Health and Greater Ability.* New York. 1882.

Holcombe, William Henry. *The Sexes Here and Hereafter.* Philadelphia, 1862.

Hollick, Frederick. *The Male Generative Organs, in Health and Disease, From Infancy to Old Age*. New York, 1855.

——. *The Marriage Guide or Natural History of Generation; A private instructor for married persons and those about to marry, both male and female*. 200th ed. New York, 1860.

——. *The Nerves and the Nervous. A practical treatise on the anatomy and physiology of the nervous system*. New York, 1873.

——. *Neuropathy; or, The true principles of the art of healing the sick. Being an explanation of the action of galvanism, electricity, and magnetism, in the cure of disease*. Philadelphia, 1847.

Hooker, Mrs. Isabella (Beecher). *Womanhood: Its Sanctities and Fidelities*. Boston, 1873.

Hor and Sprague. "Nymphomania," *Boston Medical and Surgical Journal*, 25 (1841-1842): 61.

Ingersoll, Andrew J. *In Health*. Corning, N.Y., 1878.

Isaacs, Charles Edward. "Peculiar Cerebral Symptoms Depending Upon Excessive Sexual Indulgence," *Transactions of the Medical Society of Kings County* (Brooklyn), 1 (1865): 7-9.

Jackson, James Caleb. *Dyspepsia and Its Treatment*. Dansville, N.Y., 1871.

——. *Flesh as Food for Man*. Dansville, N.Y., 1868.

——. *The Four Drunkards*. Dansville, N.Y., 1868.

——. *The Gluttony Plague; or How Persons Kill Themselves by Eating*. Dansville, N.Y., 1870.

——. *Hints on the Reproductive Organs: Their diseases, causes, and cure on hydropathic principles*. Boston and New York, 1853.

——. *How to Cure Drunkards*. Dansville, N.Y., 1868.

——. *The Sexual Organism, and Its Healthful Management*. Boston, 1861.

——. *Tobacco; and Its Effect Upon the Health and Character of Those Who Use It*. New York, 1864.

Jacobi, Abraham. "On Masturbation and Hysteria in Young Children," *American Journal of Obstetrics* (New York), 8 (1876): 595; 9: 218.

Johnston, John M. *A Treatise on the Different Forms of Venereal Disease, and on Onanism, or the Solitary Habit of Youth*. Baltimore, 1845.

Jordan, Henry J. *The Philosophy of Marriage, being eight important lectures on the functions and disorders of the nervous system, reproductive organs, and special diseases*. New York, 1863.

Kellogg, John Harvey. *First Book in Physiology and Hygiene.* New York, 1888.

——. *Ladies' Guide in Health and Disease. Girlhood, maidenhood, wifehood, motherhood.* Des Moines, 1883.

——. *The physical, moral and social effects of alcoholic poison as a beverage and as a medicine.* Battle Creek, Mich., 1876.

——. *Plain Facts about Sexual Life.* Battle Creek, Mich., 1877.

——. *Rational Hydrotherapy.* Battle Creek, Mich., 1900.

——. *Text-book of anatomy, physiology, and hygiene.* Battle Creek, Mich., 1881.

——. *The Uses of Water in Health and Disease. A practical treatise on the bath, its history and uses.* Battle Creek, Mich., 1876.

Kent, Austin. *Free Love: or, A philosophical demonstration of the non-exclusive nature of connubial love, also, a review of the exclusive feature of the Fowlers, Adin Ballou, H. C. Wright, and Andrew Jackson Davis on marriage.* Hopkinton, N.Y., 1857.

Kent, James Tyler, *Sexual Neuroses.* St. Louis, 1879.

Knowlton, Charles. *The Fruits of Philosophy; or, the private companion of young married people.* New York, 1832.

Lallemand, (Claude) François. *A Practical Treatise on the Causes, Symptoms, and Treatment of Spermatorrhoea.* Philadelphia, 1848.

——. *On Involuntary Seminal Discharges.* Philadelphia, 1839.

Larmont, Martin. *Medical Advisor and Marriage Guide, Representing all the diseases of the genital organs of the male and female.* New York, 1859.

Lazarus, M. Edgeworth. *The Human Trinity; or, Three Aspects of Life: the passional, the intellectual, the practical sphere.* New York, 1851.

——. *Involuntary Seminal Losses: their causes, effects, and cure.* New York, 1852.

——. *Love versus Marriage.* New York, 1852.

——. *Passional Hygiene and Natural Medicine; embracing the harmonies of man with his planet.* New York, 1852.

Lewis, Dio, *Chastity: or, Our Secret Sins.* New York, 1874.

——. *Five-minute Chats with Young Women, and Certain Other Parties.* New York, 1874.

——. *Our Digestion; or My Jolly Friend's Secret.* New York, 1872.

——. *Our Girls.* New York, 1871.

——. *Talks about Other People's Stomachs.* Boston, 1870.

Licentiousness, and its effects upon bodily and mental health.
New York, 1844.

Long, J. A. "A Case of Onanism; presenting great difficulty of diagnosis,"
Southern Medical and Surgical Journal (Augusta), 8 (1852): 208-210.

"Masturbation," *Boston Medical and Surgical Journal*, 27 (1842-1843),
102-108.

McMinn, S. N. "Insanity cured by excision of the external organs of
generation," *Boston Medical and Surgical Journal* 32 (1845): 131.

Miller, C. B. "Masturbation," *American Practitioner* (Louisville), 15
(1877): 281-286.

Miller, Eli Peck. *Dyspepsia: its varieties, causes, symptoms, and treatment by hydropathy and hygiene.* New York, 1870.

——. *A Father's Advice; A Book for Every Boy.* New York, 1881.

——. *A Treatise on the Cause of Exhausted Vitality; or, Abuses of the
sexual function.* New York, 1867.

Miller, Nancy Minerva [Mrs. Eli Peck]. *A Mother's Advice: A Book for
every girl.* New York, 1870.

Miller, T. "Precocious Masturbation," *National Medical Journal* (Washington), 2 (1871-1872): 355.

Napheys, George H. *The Physical Life of Women: Advice to the Maiden,
Wife and Mother.* Philadelphia, 1869.

——. *The Transmission of Life. Counsels of the nature and hygiene of the
masculine function.* Philadelphia, 1871.

Newton, Alonzo Eliot. *The Better Way: an appeal to men in behalf of human culture through a wiser parentage.* New York, 1875.

Neyman, E. H. "A Case of Masturbation," *Chicago Medical Examiner* 3
(1862): 523-531.

Nichols, Mary Gove. *Experience in Water Cure.* New York, 1850.

——. *Lectures to Ladies on Anatomy and Physiology.* Boston, 1842.

Nichols, Thomas Low. *Esoteric Anthropology: A Comprehensive and
Confidential Treatise on the Structure, Functions, Passional Attractions and Perversions, True and False Physical and Social Conditions,
and the Most Intimate Relations of Men and Women.* New York, 1853.

——. *An Introduction to the Water-Cure. A Concise Exposition of the
Human Constitution, the Conditions of Health, etc. Founded in Nature
and Adapted to the Wants of Man.* New York, 1850.

Nichols, Thomas Low and Mary Gove Nichols. *Marriage: Its History,
Character, and Results.* Cincinnati, 1854.

——. *Nichols' Medical Miscellanies; A Familiar Guide to the Preservation of Health, and the Hydropathic Home Treatment of the Most Formidable Diseases.* Cincinnati, 1856.

Nicholson, Mrs. Asenath. *Nature's Own Book.* Boston, 1835.

Noyes, John Humphrey. *Male Continence, or Self-Control in Sexual Intercourse.* Oneida, 1872.

Pancoast, Seth. *The Ladies' Medical Guide and Marriage Friend. . . .* Philadelphia, 1859.

——. *Onanism: Spermatorrhoea; Porneio-kalogynomia-pathology; Boyhood's perils and Manhood's Curse. An earnest appeal to the Young of America.* Philadelphia, 1858.

Payne, R. L. "A Case of Nymphomania," *Medical Journal of North Carolina* (Raleigh), 1-2 (1858-1859): 569.

Pendleton, Mrs. Hester. *Husband and Wife; or, the Science of Human Development Through Inherited Tendencies.* New York, 1863.

——. *The Parents' guide for the Transmission of Desired Qualities to Offspring; and Childbirth Made Easy.* New York, 1848.

Pierce, Ray Vaughn. *The People's Common Sense Medical Advisor in Plain English; or, Medicine Simplified.* Buffalo, 1875.

Pomeroy, S. F. "A Case of Masturbation, Successfully Treated by Tying the Spermatic Arteries," *Boston Medical and Surgical Journal* 52 (1869): 184.

Pope, B. A. "Opium as a Tonic and Alternative; with Remarks upon the Hypodermic Use of the Sulphate of Morphia, and its Use in the Debility and Amaurosis Consequent upon Onanism," *New Orleans Medical and Surgical Journal* 2 (1869): 184.

Porter. *Book of Men, Women, and Babies. The Laws of God Applied to Obtaining, Rearing, and Developing the Natural, Healthful, and Beautiful in Humanity. Forming a Compendium on Baby Conventions, Prize Babies, Species of Beauty; Marriage in its Varied Relations; Conception, Generation, Parturition, Transmission; Choice of Lovers, Husbands, Wives; Temperaments for Pairs; Influences of Clime, Season, Ailment, and Dress on Health and Energy; Beauty of Features increased; Weaknesses Strengthened; Defects Supplied; Faculties Legitimately Used; Laws of Exercise, Grace, Growth, Posture, Sleep, and Every Practical Instruction, For Promoting Happiness and Beautiful Babies.* New York, 1855.

Purple, William D. "On the Morbid Condition of the Generative Organs," *New York Journal of Medicine* 3 (1849): 207-218.
Root, Harmon Knox. *The Lover's Marriage Lighthouse; A Series of Sensible and Scientific Essays on the Subjects of Marriage and Free Divorce, and on the Use, Wants, and Supplies of the Spiritual, Intellectual, Affectional, and Sexual Natures of Man and Woman; Being a Key to the Causes, Prevention, Remedies, and Cure of Mental and Physical Uncongenialities Pertaining to the Indissoluble Matrimonial Institution with Original and Interesting Treaties on Love, Sexuality, Female Self-Pollution, Onanism, Attraction and Repulsion of the Sexes, Virginity, Technical Virtue, Various Customs of Marriage and Copulation, Freedom of Marriage, Divorce, Matrimonial Advertising, Noctural Emissions, Legal Marriage, Union without Law, Divinity of Sexuality, Prostitution from Indissoluble Marriage, Sickness from Uncongenial Unions, Affectional and Passional Attraction, Physiological Incest, No Seduction without Consent, etc., With Much Valuable Information and some New Views Upon the Origin and Care of Various Diseases; also, the Marriage and Divorce Laws of the Several States.* New York, 1858.
Shew, Joel. *Children, Their Hydropathic Management in Health and Disease.* New York, 1852.
——. *Tobacco: Its History, Nature and Effects on the Body and Mind.* New York, 1849.
——. *The Water-Cure Manual.* New York, 1848.
Shew, Mary Louise. *Water-Cure for Ladies.* New York, 1844.
Sizer, Nelson. *Cupid's Eyes Opened and Mirror of Matrimony in Two Lectures Originally Delivered at the Medical College, Washington, D.C., May, 1841.* Hartford, Conn., 1848.
——. *Thoughts on Domestic Life; or Marriage Vindicated and Free Love Exposed.* New York, 1848.
Storer, Horatio Robinson. "A Case of Nymphomania," *American Journal of Medical Science* (Philadelphia), 32 (1856): 378-387.
——. "Nymphomania; Removal of Foreign Bodies from the Bladder," *Boston Medical and Surgical Journal,* 60 (1856-1857): 210.
——. "On Self-Abuse in Women; Its Causation and Rational Treatment," *Western Journal of Medicine* (Indianapolis), 2 (1867): 449-457.
Swedenborg, Emanuel. *Conjugal Love and Its Chaste Delights.* New York, 1846.

Taliaferro, Valentine H. "Case of Infantile Masturbation," *Atlanta Medical and Surgical Journal* 15 (1877-1878): 460-464.

Taylor, Walter C. *A Physician's Counsels to Man in Health and Disease.* Springfield, Mass., 1872.

——. *A Physician's Counsels to Woman, In Health and Disease.* Springfield, Mass., 1872.

Tissot, Samuel A. A. D. *A Discourse on Onanism.* New York, 1832.

Trall, Russell Thacher. *Digestion and Dyspepsia; a Complete Explanation of the Physiology of the Digestive Process with the Symptoms and Treatment of Dyspepsia and other Disorders of the Digestive Organs.* New York, 1874.

——. *Home-Treatment for Sexual Abuses. A Practical Treatise on the Nature and Causes of Excessive and Unnatural Sexual Indulgence, The Diseases and Injuries Resulting Therefrom, With Their Symptoms and Hydropathic Management.* New York, 1853.

——. *The Hydropathic Encyclopedia: A System of Hydropathy and Hygiene.* New York, 1851.

——. *The Hygienic System.* Battle Creek, Mich., 1872.

——. *Nervous Debility; The Nature, Causes, Consequences, and Hygienic Treatment of Invalids Suffering From Prematurely Exhausted Vitality.* New York, 1861.

——. *The New Hydropathic Cookbook; With Recipes for Cooking on Hygienic Principles.* New York, 1853.

——. *Pathology of the Reproductive Organs, Embracing All Forms of Sexual Disorders.* Boston, 1861.

——. *Sexual Physiology; A Scientific and Popular Exposition of the Fundamental Problems in Sociology.* New York, 1866.

Wakely, Robert. *Woman and Her Secret Passions; Containing an Exact Description of the Female Organs of Generation; Their Uses and Abuses; Together with a Detailed Account of the Causes and Cure of the Solitary Vice.* New York, 1846.

Walker, Alexander. *Intermarriage: Or, The Mode in Which, and the Causes Why, Beauty, Health, and Intellect Result from Certain Unions, and Deformity, Disease, and Insanity, from Others.* New York, 1839.

——. *Woman Physiologically Considered, as to Mind, Morals, Marriage, Matrimonial Slavery, Infidelity, and Divorce.* New York, 1840.

Walton, J. T. "Case of Nymphomania Successfully Treated," *American Journal of Medical Science* (Philadelphia), 33 (1857): 47-50.

Ware, John. *Hints to Young Men, on the True Relation of the Sexes . . . Prepared at the Request of a Committee. . . .* Boston, 1850.

Wells, Samuel. *Wedlock; or, The Right Relations of the Sexes: Disclosing the Laws of Conjugal Selection, and Showing Who May, and Who May Not Marry.* New York, 1869.

Whitmore, J. S. "Venereal Excess, With Mental Impairment," *Chicago Medical Journal* 27 (1870): 23-27.

Willard, Mrs. Elizabeth Osgood Goodrich. *Sexology as the Philosophy of Life: Implying Social Organization and Government.* Chicago, 1867.

Woodward, Samuel Bayard. *Hints for the Young, on a Subject Relating to the Health of Body and Mind. From the Boston Medical and Surgical Journal, With Additions by the Author.* Boston and Worcester, 1838.

———. "Remarks on Masturbation," *Boston Medical and Surgical Journal* 12 (1835): 109, 138.

Wright, Henry Clarke. *The Empire of the Mother Over the Character and Destiny of the Race.* Boston, 1863.

———. *Marriage and Parentage; or, The Reproductive Element in Man as a Means to His Elevation and Happiness.* Boston, 1855.

———. *The Unwelcome Child; or the Crime of an Undesigned and Undesired Maternity.* Boston, 1858.

Young, William. *Marriage. Pocket Aesculapius; or, Every one His own Physician; Being Observations on Marriage, Medically and Philosophically Considered, as Manhood's Early Decline, with Directions for its Perfect Cure, etc.* Philadelphia, 1848.

Youman [pseud.]. *Dr. Youman's Illustrated Marriage Guide and Confidential Medical Advisor; A Practical Treatise on the Uses and Abuses of the Generative Functions.* Williamsburgh, N.Y., 1876.

SEXUAL HYGIENE LITERATURE PUBLISHED IN AMERICA AND ENGLAND BEFORE 1830

Because the pre-1830 literature on this subject is so scanty, I have chosen to put it in a separate list, and to include works printed in England as well as the United States. Except for *Onania*, Cotton Mather's *Pure*

Nazarite, and one article from a medical journal, none of the items on this list was ever printed in America.

Buchan, Alexander Peter. *Venus Sine Concubitu.* London, 1822.

Caton, Thomas Mott. *Practical observations on the debilities, natural and contracted, of the generative organs of both sexes.* 2nd ed. London, 1812.

———. *A practical treatise on the prevention and cure of the venereal disease . . . with some strictures on onanism.* 4th ed. London, 1811.

An Essay, addressed to all parents, guardians, and teachers, as well as to all orders of medical men, upon a vice, the bane of the moral and physical constitution of the youthful of both sexes. By a well-wisher to mankind. London, 1824.

Defoe, Daniel. *Conjugal Lewdness; Or, Matrimonial Whoredom [A Treatise concerning the Use and Abuse of the Marriage Bed].* London, 1727.

Farrer, William. *A Short Treatise on Onanism, or the detestable vice of self-pollution. Describing the varieties of nervous and other disorders that are occasioned by that shameful practice, or too early and excessive venery, and directing the best method for their cure.* 2nd ed. London, 1767.

Graham, James. *A New and Curious Treatise. . . . To which is added an appendix containing pathetic remonstrances and advices to young persons, and to old men, against the abuse of certain debilitating and degrading pleasures.* London, 1793.

Hodson, James. *Nature's assistant to the restoration of health; to which is added, a short treatise on the venereal disease; also an essay on gleets, seminal weaknesses, and a destructive habit of a private nature.* 11th ed. London, 1785.

Mather, Cotton. *The Pure Nazarite.* Boston, 1723.

Onanism Display'd; being, I. An enquiry into the true nature of Onan's sin. II. Of the modern onanists. III. Of self-pollution, its causes and consequences; with three extraordinary cases, of two young gentlemen and a lady, who were very much addicted to this crime. IV. Of nocturnal-pollutions natural and forc'd. V. The great sin of self-pollution, with the judgment of the most eminent divines upon this subject. VI. A dissertation concerning generation; with a curious description of the parts, and of their proper functions, etc., according to the latest, and most approv'd, anatomical discoveries. Translated from the Paris edition. 2nd ed. London, 1719.

Onania, or the heinous sin of self-pollution, and all its frightful consequences in both sexes considered. 10th ed. Boston, 1724.

Smyth, J. H. *A New Treatise on the Venereal Disease, Gleets, Seminal Weaknesses; the dreadful effects of self-pollution, and the causes of impotency, barrenness, etc.; directing methods of cure, established by repeated experience.* London, 1773.

A Supplement to the Onania. 20th ed. Glasgow, after 1742.

Tabes Dorsalis, or The cause of consumption in young men and women, with an explication of its symptoms, precautions, and the methods of cure; to which is added a physical account of the nature and effects of venery, as far as relates to young men, etc., its use and abuse, when and in what circumstances salutory or pernicious to persons of different ages, temperaments, and constitutions. London, 1758.

Tissot, Samuel A. A. D. *Onanism: or, A treatise upon the disorders produced by masturbation: or, the dangerous effects of secret and excessive venery.* London, 1766.

Tully, William. "An Instance of Death from Onanism," *Transactions of the Physiological Medical Society of New York* 1 (1817): 321-326.

INDEX